Eternal Energy

Superfoods for Longevity

By
Dr. Noah Wellington

Eternal Energy

Superfoods for Longevity

Table of Contents

Introduction

Welcome to a journey of vibrant health and extended longevity through the power of nutrient-rich superfoods. Our modern diets, often laden with processed foods and lacking essential nutrients, contribute to a range of health issues, from chronic diseases to diminished vitality. But there is a way to reclaim our health and well-being: incorporating superfoods into our daily lives.

In this book, we aim to demystify the world of superfoods, offering practical guidance on how to enrich your diet with these nutritional powerhouses. Whether you're new to the concept of superfoods or looking to deepen your understanding, this guide provides the knowledge and tools necessary to make informed dietary choices.

Superfoods are more than just a trendy topic; they are scientifically validated sources of vital nutrients that can support overall well-being. From antioxidant-rich fruits and leafy greens to wholesome grains and potent spices, these foods have unique properties that can enhance your body's ability to function optimally. By understanding and embracing superfoods, we can make significant strides toward better health.

Our approach is grounded in both science and practical application. You'll find detailed explanations of the nutritional benefits of various superfoods, alongside tips and recipes that make it easy to include them in your meals. We have structured the content to be both educational and actionable, so you can start making healthy changes right away.

Imagine starting your day with a smoothie packed with antioxidant-rich berries and leafy greens. Picture a lunch and dinner that not only satisfies your palate but also fuels your body with essential vitamins, minerals, and antioxidants. Superfoods offer a delicious and straightforward way to support your health goals, whether that's boosting immunity, enhancing energy, or promoting heart health.

Each chapter of this book delves into different categories of superfoods. We begin with an overview of what constitutes a superfood and the science that backs their health benefits. As you progress through the chapters, you'll discover specific foods that deserve a place on your plate and how to prepare them deliciously.

The wide array of superfoods means there's something for everyone. Are you a fan of fruits? Blueberries and pomegranates are waiting to be part of your dietary repertoire. Do you lean toward hearty meals? Whole grains like quinoa and brown rice are both versatile and nutritious. Even if you have a sweet tooth, we've got you covered with healthy dessert options like dark chocolate and berries with Greek yogurt.

One of the critical aspects we'll explore is how superfoods can fit into different lifestyles and dietary preferences. From vegans to meat-eaters, there are superfoods that can meet your nutritional needs while aligning with your individual preferences and values. Whether you enjoy cooking elaborate meals or prefer quick and easy snacks, you will find practical advice to suit your lifestyle.

Sustainability is another vital component of our discussion. As we embrace these nutrient-dense foods, it's important to consider their environmental impact. Sustainable farming practices and reducing food waste are key themes that we'll touch upon, ensuring that our choices benefit not just our health but the planet as well.

We also seek to clear the fog of misinformation that often surrounds superfoods. Myths and misconceptions can deter people from fully benefiting from these foods. By addressing common myths and providing evidence-based insights, we aim to equip you with the knowledge to make confident dietary choices.

The journey doesn't end with knowledge; it's about integration. Our goal is to help you seamlessly incorporate superfoods into your daily routine. From shopping tips and meal planning to preparing kid-friendly dishes, you'll find a variety of strategies to make superfoods an enjoyable and regular part of your life.

You deserve to feel your best, and superfoods are a tool to help you achieve that. The path to health and longevity is paved with choices we make every day, and choosing nutrient-rich, whole foods can profoundly impact our well-being. As you read through each chapter, we hope you'll be inspired to take practical steps toward a healthier, more vibrant life.

In conclusion, this book is not just about identifying superfoods but about empowering you to make lasting, positive changes in your diet and lifestyle. By exploring and embracing the wealth of nutrients that superfoods offer, you are taking charge of your health, one meal at a time. Let's embark on this journey together, unlocking the secrets of superfoods and transforming our lives with every bite.

Chapter 1:
Understanding Superfoods

Superfoods have captured the attention of health enthusiasts and researchers alike, spotlighting their potential to enhance overall well-being and longevity. Defined by their high nutrient density and powerful health benefits, these foods are often packed with vitamins, minerals, antioxidants, and other compounds essential for optimal health. The concept of superfoods is not just a modern trend; it's rooted in centuries of traditional medicine and culinary practices. Understanding what qualifies a food as a superfood requires a look into their nutritional profiles and the scientific research supporting their health claims. From improving heart health and brain function to boosting immunity and reducing inflammation, superfoods offer a natural approach to preventing chronic diseases and improving quality of life. By incorporating a variety of these nutrient-dense options into your daily diet, you can take significant steps toward a healthier, more vibrant life.

Defining Superfoods for Longevity

In the quest for a long, healthy life, superfoods have emerged as potent allies. But what exactly are these nutritional powerhouses? Superfoods are a category of foods that provide a broad range of essential nutrients while offering significant health benefits. They are not just about caloric content but about the quality of those calories—how they nourish the body and promote overall well-being.

To delve deeper, it's important to understand the genesis of the term "superfood." Although it has been widely popularized in recent decades, the concept has roots in traditional diets and ancient medicinal practices. Societies worldwide have long recognized the health-boosting properties of certain foods that go beyond basic nutrition. These foods often come packed with vitamins, minerals, antioxidants, and other bioactive compounds that contribute to various aspects of health.

A defining trait of superfoods is their nutrient density. Nutrient-dense foods provide substantial amounts of vitamins and minerals relative to their calorie content. For example, spinach is incredibly low in calories yet packs a wallop of vitamins A, C, and K, along with manganese, iron, and calcium. In contrast, less nutrient-dense foods provide fewer vitamins and minerals for the same calorie content, making them less effective for nutrition and longevity.

Longevity-focused superfoods often share common characteristics, such as high antioxidant levels. Antioxidants play a key role in neutralizing harmful free radicals, unstable molecules that can damage cells and contribute to aging and diseases like cancer. By including antioxidant-rich foods in your diet, you can combat oxidative stress and maintain cellular health, which supports longevity.

Another key aspect lies in the anti-inflammatory properties of many superfoods. Chronic inflammation has been linked to a plethora of age-related diseases, including heart disease, diabetes, and arthritis. Foods like turmeric, which contains the active ingredient curcumin, are sought after for their potent anti-inflammatory effects. Incorporating such foods can help mitigate inflammation and enhance your quality of life as you age.

Superfoods for longevity also often exhibit immunomodulating properties, meaning they can help regulate the immune system. For instance, medicinal mushrooms like reishi and shiitake have been found to enhance immune responses and improve resilience against infections. A robust immune system is crucial for longevity, as it enables the body to fend off illnesses that can strain our health over time.

Another defining factor is the presence of bioactive compounds that improve metabolic functions. Some superfoods contain phytonutrients that stimulate metabolic processes, helping the body efficiently manage energy and ward off metabolic syndrome, a cluster of conditions that increase the risk of heart disease and diabetes. Quinoa, chia seeds, and other whole grains offer complex carbohydrates and fibers that stabilize blood sugar levels, thus supporting metabolic health.

Beyond the physical benefits, superfoods can positively impact psychological health, which is paramount for longevity. Foods rich in omega-3 fatty acids, such as salmon and flaxseeds, contribute to brain health by supporting cognitive function and reducing the risk of neurodegenerative diseases like Alzheimer's. A well-nourished brain is crucial for maintaining mental acuity and emotional balance as we age.

However, not all superfoods are created equal, and their impacts can vary based on factors such as how they're grown, processed, and consumed. It's essential to prioritize organic and minimally-processed options to maximize their health benefits. Nutrient degradation can occur when foods are overly processed or exposed to pesticides and other chemicals, reducing their effectiveness.

Integrating superfoods into daily life doesn't have to be complicated or expensive. Many superfoods are accessible and versatile, fitting seamlessly into various diets. For example, incorporating berries, leafy greens, and nuts into your meals can be as simple as adding a handful of blueberries to your breakfast oatmeal, tossing a mix of spinach and kale into your lunchtime salad, or snacking on a mix of almonds and seeds throughout the day.

Variety is also crucial. While it's easy to latch onto a single "super" ingredient, a diverse diet rich in different superfoods will provide a broad spectrum of nutrients that support holistic health. Rotating between different fruits, vegetables, whole grains, and proteins ensures you cover all your nutritional bases.

It's worthwhile to consider the cultural and culinary joys of superfoods as well. Many of these nutrient-rich foods have distinct flavors and textures that can transform your culinary experiences. Experimenting with recipes from different cultures can not only diversify your palate but also enrich your nutrient intake. The global pantry of superfoods—ranging from the quinoa of South America to the turmeric of India—offers endless culinary and health possibilities.

As you start integrating superfoods into your routine, portion control and balance remain essential. Even nutrient-dense foods, when consumed in excess, can lead to imbalances or unwanted calories. Approaching superfoods with mindfulness, as part of a balanced diet, will support sustained health benefits rather than short-term gains.

The science supporting superfoods is constantly evolving, but the consensus remains clear: foods rich in essential nutrients and bioactive compounds can significantly impact health and longevity. Staying informed about ongoing research can help you make educated choices about which foods to prioritize for your unique health goals. Reliable sources and expert advice can provide insights into tailoring superfood choices to individual needs, ensuring you're always on the path to optimal health.

In summary, defining superfoods for longevity involves recognizing these foods' dense nutritional profiles and their potential to fortify the body against age-related conditions. These foods offer a robust suite of health benefits, from antioxidants and anti-inflammatory agents to immune boosters and metabolic enhancers. By incorporating a diverse array of superfoods into your daily diet, you lay a strong foundation for long-lasting health and vitality.

The Science Behind Nutrient-Dense Foods

When delving into the world of superfoods, it becomes essential to understand what makes certain foods so exceptionally good for you. The term "nutrient-dense" refers to foods that provide a high concentration of vitamins, minerals, and other health-promoting components in relation to their calorie content. But what exactly constitutes this nutrient density, and how can it influence your journey towards improved health and longevity?

One of the fundamental elements behind nutrient-dense foods lies in their assortment of vitamins. Vitamins are organic compounds that your body needs in small amounts to function correctly. They facilitate numerous biochemical processes; for example, Vitamin C is essential for the synthesis of collagen, while Vitamin A is crucial for vision and immune function. Nutrient-dense superfoods often contain multiple vitamins that work synergistically to bolster your health.

Minerals like calcium, magnesium, and potassium also play a crucial role in nutrient-dense foods. These inorganic elements are necessary for various bodily functions, ranging from muscle contraction to nerve function to bone health. Foods rich in these minerals provide substantial benefits while also contributing crucially to overall well-being. For instance, the potassium found in leafy greens helps to regulate blood pressure, an essential component for cardiovascular health.

Phytochemicals are another exceptional component of nutrient-dense foods. These naturally occurring chemical compounds are found in plants and have been shown to offer various health benefits. These include antioxidants, flavonoids, and polyphenols, which help fight chronic diseases and support long-term health. Phytochemicals work along with vitamins and minerals to offer a comprehensive range of health benefits. Blueberries, rich in anthocyanins, have been shown to improve cognitive function and reduce inflammation.

The macronutrient profile of food—carbohydrates, proteins, and fats—is another aspect that contributes to nutrient density. While many people focus solely on calorie content, the quality of these macronutrients matters. Whole grains like quinoa offer complex carbohydrates that provide sustained energy and fiber, aiding digestion. Fatty fish like salmon supply omega-3 fatty acids, which are crucial for heart and brain health. Meanwhile, proteins from legumes and nuts support muscle repair and growth. This balanced macronutrient content adds to the overall nutrient density of the food.

Antioxidants are particularly noteworthy when discussing nutrient-dense foods. These molecules inhibit oxidation, a chemical reaction that can produce free radicals leading to cell damage. Antioxidants neutralize free radicals, thereby preventing or slowing damage to cells. Foods rich in antioxidants, such as berries and dark leafy greens, are vital for protecting against a myriad of diseases, including cancer and heart disease. The synergistic action of antioxidants with other nutrients boosts the overall efficacy of these superfoods.

Moreover, dietary fiber found in many nutrient-dense foods supports digestive health. It adds bulk to the stool, facilitating regular bowel movements and preventing constipation. But fiber does more than aid digestion. It helps to regulate blood sugar levels by slowing the absorption of sugar into the bloodstream, which is particularly beneficial for individuals managing diabetes. Additionally, fiber can assist in weight control as it promotes a feeling of fullness, discouraging overeating.

Micronutrients also play an integral part in the nutrient profiles of superfoods. Though required in smaller amounts, micronutrients like iron, zinc, and selenium perform crucial functions. Iron is essential for transporting oxygen in your blood; zinc supports immune function, and selenium acts as a powerful antioxidant. Foods like spinach, nuts, and seeds are packed with these micronutrients, offering significant health advantages with minimal calorie intake.

Other components like enzymes and healthy fatty acids can contribute to the nutrient density of a food. Enzymes help catalyze biochemical reactions in the body, such as digestion and metabolism. Raw veggies are rich in these enzymes, which can be destroyed during cooking. Healthy fatty acids, such as those found in avocado and olive oil, play a crucial role in cell membrane integrity and hormone production. These additional elements add to the robust nutritional profile of superfoods.

A decidedly significant concept is bioavailability, which refers to how well your body can absorb and utilize the nutrients in a food. Just because a food is high in nutrients doesn't mean your body can access all those nutrients. Factors like the presence of other nutrients, food preparation methods, and individual health conditions can influence bioavailability. For example, the iron in meat (heme iron) is more readily absorbed by the body than the iron in spinach (non-heme iron). Similarly, cooking tomatoes increases the bioavailability of lycopene, a powerful antioxidant.

The manner in which food is grown, harvested, and prepared can impact its nutrient density. Organic farming practices, often touted for environmental benefits, can also result in higher nutrient content. Rotating crops and using compost can increase the mineral content of the soil, which in turn elevates the nutritional profile of the plants grown in it. Similarly, consuming foods fresh and minimally processed preserves their nutrient content. Freezing, canning, and other preservation methods can lead to nutrient loss, meaning fresh or lightly cooked foods tend to be more nutrient-dense.

Incorporating a variety of nutrient-dense foods into your diet ensures you get a comprehensive range of essential nutrients. Diversity in your diet not only prevents nutrient deficiencies but also maximizes the health benefits you gain from different foods. A blend of colorful fruits, leafy greens, whole grains, and lean proteins can cover all bases, offering a wide array of vitamins, minerals, and other beneficial compounds. Meal planning and smart shopping can help make this diverse, nutrient-dense diet more achievable.

Lastly, the role of nutrient-dense foods in disease prevention cannot be overstated. Chronic diseases such as heart disease, diabetes, and cancer are often linked to poor diet choices. A nutrient-dense diet helps protect against these ailments. Foods rich in antioxidants, healthy fats, and anti-inflammatory compounds bolster your body's defense mechanisms, enhancing your longevity and quality of life. By focusing on nutrient-dense foods, you set a strong foundation for lifelong health.

The science behind nutrient-dense foods reveals that they are not just a trendy concept but a cornerstone of health and longevity. With their rich profile of vitamins, minerals, phytochemicals, and other beneficial compounds, nutrient-dense foods offer an array of advantages that can support and elevate your well-being. By understanding the underlying science, you can make informed choices that enrich your dietary habits and, consequently, your life.

Chapter 2:
Antioxidant-Rich Fruits

Antioxidant-rich fruits are nature's powerful allies in our quest for health and longevity, packed with compounds that combat oxidative stress and reduce inflammation. These fruits, such as blueberries and pomegranates, are not only delicious but also brimming with vitamins, minerals, and phytonutrients essential for maintaining robust health. Blueberries, often dubbed the "antioxidant powerhouse," offer a delightful way to support brain function and heart health. Pomegranates, with their deep ruby seeds, have been cherished since ancient times for their potent anti-inflammatory properties and ability to enhance cardiovascular health. Incorporating these fruits into your daily diet can help you harness their protective benefits, whether enjoyed fresh, blended into smoothies, or sprinkled over a vibrant salad. Embracing the habitual consumption of these antioxidant-packed fruits not only satisfies the palate but also fortifies the body against the wear and tear of daily life.

Blueberries: The Antioxidant Powerhouse

Blueberries truly live up to their reputation as an antioxidant powerhouse, packing an impressive punch of nutrients in every small bite. These vibrant berries are loaded with vitamins C and K, fiber, and a range of phytonutrients, making them one of the top choices for boosting overall health. Thanks to their high levels of anthocyanins— the compounds responsible for their deep blue color—blueberries help neutralize free radicals in the body, thereby reducing oxidative stress and lowering the risk of chronic diseases like heart disease and cancer. Whether you're tossing them into a morning smoothie, mixing them into oatmeal, or enjoying them as a fresh snack, incorporating blueberries into your daily diet is a delicious way to harness their potent health benefits and give your body a robust line of defense against aging and disease.

Delicious Blueberry Recipes Blueberries, nature's little blue gems, are not only a delight to the taste buds but also a powerhouse of nutrients and antioxidants. They are incredibly versatile, seamlessly fitting into various dishes, from breakfast staples to sophisticated desserts. Whether you're a culinary novice or a seasoned cook, you'll find numerous ways to incorporate blueberries into your daily meals.

First up, let's talk about an easy and nutritious option—Blueberry Overnight Oats. This recipe is perfect for busy mornings or those looking to jumpstart their day with a nutrient-filled meal. Combine 1/2 cup rolled oats, 1/2 cup almond milk, 1/2 cup Greek yogurt, and 1/2 cup fresh or frozen blueberries in a mason jar. Stir well, seal, and refrigerate overnight. In the morning, give it another stir and top with a handful of nuts or a drizzle of honey. This simple dish not only satisfies but also ensures you get a good dose of antioxidants, fiber, and protein.

If you prefer something warm and comforting, Blueberry Pancakes are a fantastic choice. Start by whisking together 1 cup all-purpose flour, 1 tablespoon sugar, 1 teaspoon baking powder, and 1/2 teaspoon salt. In another bowl, mix 1 cup milk, 1 egg, and 2 tablespoons melted butter. Combine the wet and dry ingredients, adding 1 cup fresh blueberries just before pouring spoonfuls of the batter onto a hot, greased griddle. Cook until bubbles form on the surface, then flip and cook until both sides are golden. Top with a sprinkle of powdered sugar or a pour of pure maple syrup for an irresistible breakfast treat.

For a lunch that feels gourmet but is remarkably simple to prepare, try a Blueberry Spinach Salad. Toss together a mix of fresh spinach leaves, 1/2 cup fresh blueberries, crumbled goat cheese, and a handful of toasted walnuts. Drizzle with a homemade dressing made from 2 tablespoons olive oil, 1 tablespoon balsamic vinegar, and a teaspoon of honey. The result is a salad bursting with flavor and nutrients, perfect for a light yet satisfying meal.

Moving on to dinner, consider a Grilled Chicken with Blueberry Balsamic Glaze. The glaze is the star here, made by simmering 1/2 cup balsamic vinegar with 1 cup blueberries, 1 tablespoon honey, and a pinch of salt until it reduces to a thick, syrupy consistency. Grill your seasoned chicken breasts until cooked through, then brush generously with the blueberry balsamic glaze and serve with a side of roasted vegetables or quinoa. This dish not only impresses in flavor but also offers a unique way to include blueberries in your savory recipes.

No culinary journey with blueberries would be complete without dessert. A Blueberry Crumble is a crowd-pleaser that's both easy to make and deeply satisfying. Preheat your oven to 350°F (175°C). In a baking dish, combine 4 cups of blueberries, 1/4 cup sugar, 1 tablespoon lemon juice, and 2 tablespoons cornstarch. In a separate bowl, blend together 1 cup rolled oats, 1/2 cup all-purpose flour, 1/2 cup brown sugar, and 1/2 cup melted butter until crumbly. Sprinkle the crumble mixture evenly over the blueberries and bake for about 30 minutes or until the topping is golden brown. Serve warm, perhaps with a scoop of vanilla ice cream for added decadence.

For a refreshingly different approach, try making a Blueberry Sorbet. This frozen treat is perfect for hot days and surprisingly simple to make. Blend together 4 cups frozen blueberries, 1/2 cup sugar, and 1/4 cup freshly squeezed lemon juice until smooth. Strain the mixture to remove any solids, then pour it into an ice cream maker according to the manufacturer's instructions. If you don't have an ice cream maker, pour the mixture into a shallow dish and freeze, stirring every 30 minutes until it reaches a sorbet-like consistency. This vibrant, naturally sweetened dessert is both delicious and packed with antioxidants.

If you enjoy baking, then Blueberry Muffins might be right up your alley. These are perfect for a quick breakfast or a handy snack. Start by preheating your oven to 375°F (190°C) and lining a muffin tin with paper liners. In a large bowl, mix 1 1/2 cups all-purpose flour, 3/4 cup sugar, 1/2 teaspoon salt, and 2 teaspoons baking powder. In another bowl, combine 1/3 cup vegetable oil, 1 egg, and 1/3 cup milk. Mix the wet ingredients into the dry until just combined, then fold in 1 cup blueberries. Fill the muffin cups about two-thirds full and bake for 20-25 minutes or until a toothpick inserted into the center comes out clean. Enjoy these muffins fresh out of the oven or freeze for a quick snack later.

For those interested in something a bit more sophisticated, a Blueberry Lemon Cheesecake can capture your fancy. Begin with the crust by mixing 1 1/2 cups graham cracker crumbs with 1/4 cup melted butter. Press the mixture into the bottom of a springform pan and chill while preparing the filling. Beat together 3 packages of softened cream cheese, 1 cup sugar, and 1 teaspoon vanilla extract until smooth. Add 3 eggs, one at a time, followed by 1/4 cup fresh lemon juice and the zest of one lemon. Pour the filling over the crust and bake at 325°F (160°C) for about 55 minutes or until the center is set. Once cooled, top with a homemade blueberry sauce made by simmering 2 cups blueberries with 1/2 cup sugar and 1 tablespoon lemon juice until thickened. This dessert is a beautiful centerpiece for any occasion and tastes as good as it looks.

Even drinks can get a delicious blueberry makeover. A Blueberry Smoothie is an effortless way to infuse your day with vitamins and minerals. Blend together 1 cup frozen blueberries, 1/2 banana, 1 cup Greek yogurt, 1/2 cup spinach (optional), and 1/2 cup almond milk until smooth. This nutrient-packed drink is perfect for breakfast or as an afternoon pick-me-up. It's refreshing, filling, and incredibly good for you.

If you're in the mood for a more indulgent beverage, a Blueberry Mojito might be in order. Muddle a handful of fresh blueberries with 2 tablespoons sugar and a few fresh mint leaves at the bottom of a glass. Add the juice of one lime and 2 ounces of white rum, then fill the glass with ice. Top with club soda and give it a good stir. This cocktail is fruit-forward and refreshing, ideal for a summer gathering or a quiet evening on the porch.

From breakfast to dessert, and everything in between, blueberries offer a wealth of delicious possibilities. Remember that these recipes are just a starting point. Feel free to experiment and adjust them to your taste preferences

Pomegranate: The Ancient Superfood

Steeped in history and revered across cultures, pomegranate earns its title as an "ancient superfood" for good reason. This vibrant fruit, known for its jewel-like seeds, is not only rich in taste but also packed with potent antioxidants. Pomegranates contain high levels of vitamin C, potassium, and polyphenols that combat oxidative stress and inflammation, making them a powerhouse for boosting heart health, improving memory, and even supporting joint function. By integrating pomegranate into your daily diet, you can enjoy its unique health benefits while adding a tangy-sweet flavor to your meals. Whether you sprinkle the seeds onto salads, blend them into smoothies, or simply enjoy them on their own, pomegranate offers a versatile and delicious way to improve your antioxidant intake and overall wellness.

Integrating Pomegranate into Your Diet is one of the easiest and most rewarding steps you can take towards enriching your intake of antioxidant-rich superfoods. Pomegranate is a versatile fruit that can seamlessly become part of your daily meals, thanks to its juicy, tangy seeds that pack a delightful punch. Whether you're aiming to snack smarter or elevate the nutrient profile of your favorite dishes, pomegranates offer a simple and tasty solution.

One of the simplest ways to integrate pomegranate into your diet is by adding the seeds, or arils, to your morning routine. Sprinkle them over a bowl of oatmeal, yogurt, or even a smoothie bowl. This not only adds a burst of flavor but also provides a significant antioxidant boost to kickstart your day. You can easily prepare a week's worth of pomegranate seeds in advance, storing them in an airtight container in the refrigerator for a refreshing, convenient topping.

If you're into juicing, pomegranate juice is another fantastic option. Freshly squeezed pomegranate juice can be consumed on its own or mixed with other fruit juices to create a nutritious cocktail. It's worth noting that commercially available pomegranate juices often include added sugars and preservatives, so making your own ensures you're getting a pure, unadulterated form of this superfood. Just remember, a little goes a long way, considering its high concentration of nutrients and natural sugars.

Salads are another excellent avenue to explore when it comes to incorporating pomegranate. Toss a handful of pomegranate seeds into your salads for a sweet and tangy twist that pairs well with greens, nuts, and cheese. A spinach salad with goat cheese, walnuts, and pomegranate seeds drizzled with a balsamic vinaigrette can be both visually stunning and packed with diverse nutrients. The crunchiness of the seeds complements the softness of the spinach leaves and creaminess of the goat cheese, making each bite a balanced delight.

But don't stop at salads. Pomegranate can add flair to various savory dishes. Imagine a roasted chicken or duck glazed with a pomegranate reduction – the tartness of the pomegranate contrasts beautifully with the richness of the poultry. Or consider a Middle Eastern-inspired dish, like a lamb stew cooked with pomegranate molasses that brings a depth of flavor and complexity to the meal. The possibilities are as vast as your culinary imagination.

Beyond these straightforward approaches, pomegranate can also enhance your desserts. Pomegranate seeds can be sprinkled over ice cream, mixed into chia seed pudding, or serve as a vibrant garnish for cakes and pastries. Their bright color and contrasting texture make them a fantastic addition to any sweet treat. Moreover, they contribute significantly to the visual and nutritional appeal of desserts without the need for added refined sugar.

Another simple, yet sumptuous way to integrate pomegranate into your diet is through beverages. Pomegranate arils can be added to sparkling water or cocktails for a festive pop of color and flavor. For a more elaborate creation, try crafting a pomegranate smoothie. Blend the arils with Greek yogurt, a banana, and a handful of frozen berries for a nutrient-dense drink that can serve as a quick breakfast or a post-workout replenisher. This smoothie is loaded with antioxidants, vitamins, and protein, making it a well-rounded, energizing option.

If you're looking for a way to incorporate pomegranate flavor without the seeds, consider using pomegranate molasses. It's a thick, tangy-sweet syrup made from reduced pomegranate juice. A drizzle of pomegranate molasses can elevate an assortment of dishes – from a marinade for meats to a dressing for roasted vegetables or even as a unique topping for pancakes and waffles. This versatile condiment can be found in many grocery stores or easily made at home by simmering pomegranate juice until it achieves a molasses-like consistency.

For those with a penchant for baking, pomegranates can be a delightful ingredient in muffins, breads, and cakes. Try mixing a handful of seeds into your batter before baking. Or for a sophisticated twist, make a pomegranate glaze by mixing powdered sugar with a few tablespoons of pomegranate juice and drizzle it over cakes or scones. These small additions can transform standard recipes into something extraordinary, adding not only flavor but also a burst of beautiful ruby color.

Lastly, let's discuss the convenience factor. Pomegranate seeds are surprisingly easy to incorporate into pre-existing meal plans. You can buy whole pomegranates, remove the seeds, and freeze them for extended use. Having a bag of frozen pomegranate seeds on hand makes it easy to toss them into any dish without worrying about spoilage. This makes pomegranate a flexible and practical superfood to keep in your culinary repertoire, especially for those with busy lifestyles.

In conclusion, integrating pomegranate into your diet is not only simple but also incredibly beneficial for your health. The fruit's versatility allows it to be included in an array of meals – from breakfast to dinner, snacks to desserts. By exploring the various ways to include this superfood in your daily routine, you're taking a proactive step towards a healthier, more vibrant life. Whether you prefer its seeds, juice, or molasses form, pomegranate proves to be a delicious and nutrient-rich addition to any diet.

Chapter 3:
Leafy Greens

Stepping into the realm of leafy greens, it's clear these vibrant vegetables are indispensable in the quest for improved health and longevity. Brimming with essential vitamins, minerals, and fiber, leafy greens like kale and spinach offer a powerful punch to our daily nutrition. Imagine a bowl of kale, its dark, curly leaves packed with vitamins A, K, and C, providing a nutrient-dense foundation for salads, smoothies, and even snacks. Spinach, too, is not to be overshadowed. These tender, iron-rich leaves effortlessly blend into various dishes, making it simple to boost vitality with every meal. By incorporating these greens into your diet, you're not just adding flavor and texture; you're making a commitment to nourishing your body with the very best nature has to offer. So, as you explore the benefits of these leafy superfoods, remember that the key to longevity might just be a handful of greens away.

Kale: The Nutrient-Dense Leafy Green

Kale stands out as a powerhouse among leafy greens, offering a combination of vitamins, minerals, and antioxidants that few other plants can match. It's packed with Vitamin K, which is essential for blood clotting and bone health, and boasts high levels of Vitamin A and C to boost the immune system. Moreover, kale's dense fiber content supports digestive health and keeps you feeling full longer, making it an excellent addition to any weight management plan. Anti-inflammatory compounds in kale, such as omega-3 fatty acids and polyphenols, further elevate its status as a superfood. The glucosinolates in kale may also play a role in reducing the risk of chronic diseases, including certain cancers. Incorporating kale into your diet doesn't just add a pop of green; it contributes significantly to your overall wellness and longevity.

Cooking with Kale is an adventure into one of the most nutrient-dense leafy greens available. Kale, a superfood brimming with vitamins, minerals, antioxidants, and fiber, offers a versatile base for a variety of culinary creations. Whether you're a seasoned chef or just beginning to explore healthy eating, incorporating kale into your meals can be both simple and rewarding.

Let's start with the basics: Kale can be consumed raw, sautéed, boiled, or baked. Each method brings out unique flavors and textures that will keep your palate interested. When preparing kale, it's crucial to properly wash and de-stem the leaves. The stems are fibrous and can be a bit tough to chew, so it's best to remove them, especially if you are eating kale raw.

One of the most popular ways to enjoy kale is in salads. Raw kale can be a bit tough and bitter, but massaging the leaves with a bit of olive oil and lemon juice can transform them. This simple process softens the leaves and mellows the bitterness, resulting in a more palatable and delicious experience. Try adding a sprinkle of sea salt, some chopped nuts, and dried fruits to enhance the flavors and textures. For instance, a kale salad with cranberries, walnuts, and a light vinaigrette can be a refreshing and nutrient-packed dish.

If you're a fan of warm dishes, sautéed kale is an excellent option. Heat a pan with some olive oil and garlic, then add your kale leaves. Cook until they are wilted but still vibrant green. This method retains most of the nutrients while giving the kale a slightly nutty flavor. You can add a splash of vegetable broth or white wine for an extra layer of complexity. Sautéed kale pairs well with grains like quinoa and brown rice, which we'll explore in other chapters.

For those chilly nights, kale can be a hearty addition to soups and stews. It holds up well in simmering liquids and adds a nutritional punch to your one-pot meals. A classic kale and white bean soup is not only comforting but also packed with proteins and fibers that can keep you satisfied for hours. Just toss chopped kale into your favorite soup recipes and let it cook until tender.

Another exciting way to include kale in your diet is by baking it into kale chips. This snack is a fantastic alternative to traditional potato chips and can be customized with various seasonings. After washing and drying the kale thoroughly, toss the leaves with a small amount of olive oil and your choice of spices—think nutritional yeast for a cheesy flavor, smoked paprika for some heat, or simple sea salt. Spread the leaves in a single layer on a baking sheet and bake at a low temperature until crispy. Kale chips are a delightful way to enjoy a crunchy, guilt-free snack.

Kale can also be blended into smoothies for a nutrient boost without altering the flavor too drastically. When paired with fruits like bananas, berries, and mangoes, the slightly bitter taste of kale becomes almost undetectable. You can create green smoothies that are both delicious and nourishing. Start with a base of your favorite milk (dairy or plant-based), add a handful of fresh or frozen kale, throw in some fruits, and blend until smooth. The result is a vibrant, green drink that is as tasty as it is healthy.

Mashed potatoes, a classic comfort food, can be given a healthy twist by adding kale. Simply steam kale leaves until tender and then mash them into your cooked potatoes. This adds a pop of color and a boost of nutrients to an otherwise carb-heavy side dish. The slight texture contrast can make your mashed potatoes more interesting while sneaking in those essential vitamins and minerals.

For those who enjoy experimenting in the kitchen, kale can be creatively used in baking as well. Kale powder, made by dehydrating and grinding kale leaves, can be added to bread, muffins, and even pancakes for an unexpected nutritional enhancement. It's a subtle way to incorporate this superfood into your diet without altering the flavor profile of your favorite baked goods.

If you're hosting a dinner party or simply want a quick and tasty appetizer, kale can be incorporated into dips and spreads. Kale pesto is a delightful twist on the traditional basil pesto. Blend fresh kale with garlic, nuts (like walnuts or pine nuts), Parmesan cheese, olive oil, and a splash of lemon juice. This pesto can be used in various ways—spread on toast, mixed into pasta, or even dolloped on top of grilled meats and vegetables.

Another inventive way to use kale is by making a stuffed kale roll. Blanch large kale leaves and use them as wrappers for a filling made of grains, legumes, and herbs. Roll them up, secure with toothpicks, and bake with a tomato or creamy sauce. These rolls can be a unique and nutritious centerpiece for your meal.

For breakfast, consider adding kale to your classic scrambled eggs or omelets. Sauté the kale with onions or bell peppers before adding the eggs to the pan. This simple addition can elevate a standard breakfast dish into a superfood-rich meal. Pair with whole-grain toast or a side of avocado for a perfectly balanced start to your day.

Remember, the key to cooking with kale is to keep experimenting. Its versatility means there are nearly endless ways to enjoy this leafy green. As you explore the various culinary uses of kale, you'll find that each preparation method brings out different flavors and textures, making your meals more diverse and enriched with the health benefits that kale offers.

In the next section, we will delve into easy spinach recipes, another powerhouse leafy green that can complement your kale-based dishes. Combining different superfoods in your daily meals can optimize your nutrient intake and keep your diet interesting, colorful, and most importantly, healthy. Happy cooking!

Spinach: A Daily Dose of Vitality

Dive into the vibrant world of spinach, a leafy green that packs a punch when it comes to delivering vital nutrients essential for daily vitality. Brimming with vitamins A, C, and K, alongside iron, magnesium, and antioxidants, spinach supports everything from vision and bone health to immune function and muscle efficiency. It's no wonder this versatile superfood has earned a stellar reputation. Whether you're blending it into smoothies, tossing it into salads, or incorporating it into cooked dishes, making spinach a regular part of your diet is a simple yet profound step towards better health and longevity.

Easy Spinach Recipes provide a simple and accessible way to incorporate this nutrient-rich leafy green into your diet. Spinach's mild flavor and tender texture make it incredibly versatile, fitting seamlessly into an array of dishes, from smoothies to main courses. This section aims to provide easy recipes that any home cook can whip up, ensuring you get your daily dose of vitamins, minerals, and antioxidants.

Jumpstart your mornings with a refreshing *Spinach and Banana Smoothie*. To make this, blend a ripe banana, a handful of fresh spinach, a cup of almond milk, and a tablespoon of chia seeds. Not only is this smoothie quick and easy, but it's also packed with nutrients that can provide a sustained energy boost. The banana adds natural sweetness, while the spinach delivers a good dose of vitamins A, C, and K.

For a quick and nutritious lunch, consider a *Spinach and Avocado Salad*. Toss a couple of cups of fresh spinach with sliced avocado, cherry tomatoes, sliced red onions, and a handful of walnuts. For the dressing, mix olive oil, lemon juice, a touch of salt and pepper. This salad is not just colorful but also a bounty of healthy fats, antioxidants, and fiber. It's an ideal meal for those looking to keep their digestive system in check while enjoying a flavorful dish.

If you're more into soups, *Spinach and Lentil Soup* is both hearty and healthy. Start by sautéing onions, garlic, and carrots in olive oil until they are soft. Add vegetable broth, lentils, and a couple of cups of fresh spinach. Let it simmer until the lentils are tender. Season with salt, pepper, and a squeeze of lemon juice for added zest. This comforting soup is perfect for a cold day and provides a balanced mix of protein and greens.

Looking for a fulfilling dinner? *Spinach-Stuffed Chicken Breasts* are a must-try. Butterfly chicken breasts and stuff them with a mixture of sautéed spinach, garlic, and ricotta cheese. Secure with toothpicks, then sear the breasts in a pan until golden brown. Finish them off in the oven at 375°F (190°C) for 20 minutes, or until cooked through. These stuffed chicken breasts are packed with flavor and nutrients, making them a family favorite.

If you're in the mood for pasta, a *Spinach and Mushroom Alfredo* can be a delightful treat. Sauté mushrooms and garlic in a pan with a little olive oil, then add fresh spinach until it wilts. Mix in cooked pasta and a homemade Alfredo sauce made from cashew cream for a vegan option or traditional cream and Parmesan for a more classic version. This rich and creamy dish offers a delicious way to consume your greens, blending them seamlessly into a satisfying meal.

Another dinner option that's both simple and nutritious is *Spinach and Quinoa Stuffed Peppers*. Cook quinoa according to package instructions, then mix it with sautéed spinach, diced tomatoes, black beans, and a sprinkle of cumin and chili powder. Fill halved bell peppers with the mixture and bake at 375°F (190°C) for 25-30 minutes. The result is a colorful, flavor-packed dish that's also high in protein and fiber.

For a snack or side dish, consider *Spinach and Feta Stuffed Mushrooms*. Remove the stems from large button mushrooms and fill the caps with a mixture of chopped spinach, crumbled feta cheese, garlic, and breadcrumbs. Bake at 350°F (175°C) for about 15-20 minutes until the mushrooms are tender and the filling is golden. These bite-sized delights are perfect for parties or as a savory treat anytime.

When it's time for a quick dinner, an *Easy Spinach Frittata* is an excellent choice. Whisk together eggs, a splash of milk, salt, and pepper. In an oven-safe skillet, sauté spinach and onions until they are soft, then pour in the egg mixture. Once the edges start to set, transfer the skillet to a preheated oven at 350°F (175°C) and bake until the frittata is fully set. This dish is versatile and can be enjoyed hot or cold, making it perfect for any meal or as leftovers the next day.

If you enjoy baking, try a *Spinach and Cheese Savory Muffins*. These muffins combine baby spinach, cheddar cheese, and whole wheat flour to create a nutritious and portable snack. In a bowl, mix flour, baking powder, and a pinch of salt. In another bowl, whisk eggs, milk, and melted butter before stirring in the dry ingredients along with the spinach and cheese. Spoon the batter into a muffin tin and bake at 375°F (190°C) for about 20-25 minutes. These muffins are ideal for breakfast on-the-go or as a savory snack throughout the day.

For those special weekend brunches, you can't go wrong with *Spinach and Tomato Shakshuka*. This classic North African dish gets a nutrient boost with the addition of spinach. In a large skillet, heat some olive oil and sauté onions and garlic until soft. Add canned tomatoes, a pinch of cumin, paprika, and let the mixture simmer. Stir in a couple of cups of fresh spinach until wilted, then make small wells in the mixture and crack eggs into them. Cover the skillet and cook until the eggs are done to your liking. Serve with crusty bread to soak up the savory sauce. This dish is a surefire way to impress guests while providing a hearty and wholesome meal.

Spinach and Sweet Potato Hash adds a nutritious twist to a breakfast classic. Dice sweet potatoes and sauté them in olive oil until they start to soften. Add chopped spinach, bell peppers, and onions, cooking until all the vegetables are tender and slightly caramelized. Season with salt, pepper, and smoked paprika for a hint of spice. This hash pairs perfectly with scrambled or poached eggs, making it a hearty start to the day that's packed with vitamins and minerals.

No collection of spinach recipes would be complete without a classic *Spinach Dip*. Perfect for parties or as an everyday snack, this dip combines fresh spinach with Greek yogurt, garlic, lemon juice, and a touch of salt and pepper. Serve with whole grain crackers, fresh veggies, or spread it on whole wheat toast. This lighter version of a traditional favorite ensures you get all the benefits of spinach without the excess calories or fat.

Finally, end your day with a comforting bowl of *Spinach and Chickpea Curry*. Sauté onions, garlic, and ginger in a pan with some olive oil until they're soft. Add a can of chickpeas, a couple of cups of chopped spinach, and a mix of your favorite curry spices. Pour in a can of coconut milk and let the mixture simmer until it thickens. Serve over brown

Chapter 4:
Whole Grains

Whole grains are an essential part of a balanced diet, offering a myriad of health benefits that focus on longevity and overall wellness. These nutrient-rich powerhouses, such as quinoa and brown rice, provide a steady source of energy thanks to their complex carbohydrates and fiber content. Unlike refined grains, whole grains retain their nutrient-packed bran and germ, delivering an abundance of vitamins, minerals, and antioxidants. Consuming whole grains has been linked to reduced risks of chronic diseases, including heart disease, diabetes, and certain cancers. Including a variety of whole grains in your daily meals not only adds texture and flavor but also fortifies your body with essential nutrients needed for long-term health. Whether you're nourishing your body with a hearty quinoa salad or enjoying a comforting bowl of brown rice, these grains are sure to keep you feeling full and satisfied while promoting optimal health.

Quinoa: The Complete Protein

Quinoa, often hailed as a nutritional powerhouse, is an indispensable addition to your diet if you're aiming for a complete protein source. Unlike many plant-based foods, quinoa contains all nine essential amino acids, making it a rare find in the world of whole grains. This tiny seed is not just about protein; it's packed with fiber, magnesium, manganese, and a host of other vitamins and minerals that support overall health. Whether you incorporate it into a hearty salad, a warm breakfast porridge, or even a main course, quinoa offers versatility and sustenance. Adding quinoa to your meals is a simple yet impactful step toward achieving better health and longevity through nutrient-dense superfoods.

Quinoa for Breakfast, Lunch, and Dinner has quickly emerged as the hero of modern, health-conscious kitchens. And why not? With its unique nutritional profile, versatility, and ease of preparation, quinoa transcends the conventional boundaries of a typical grain. Often mistaken for a grain, quinoa is actually a seed from the Chenopodium quinoa plant. This pseudo-grain is power-packed with complete protein, fiber, vitamins, and essential minerals, making it a perfect candidate for any mealtime makeover.

For breakfast, quinoa can be a game-changer. Imagine starting your day with a hearty bowl of quinoa porridge. Rich in protein and fiber, quinoa will keep you full and satisfied throughout the morning. To prepare, simply cook quinoa in almond milk or any plant-based milk of your choice, add a dash of cinnamon, a spoonful of honey, and top it with berries and nuts. Not only does this breakfast taste delicious, but it also stabilizes your blood sugar levels, providing that steady energy you need to kickstart your day.

If you have a sweet tooth, quinoa breakfast muffins could be your new favorite. These muffins are easy to make in batches and keep for a few days. Blend cooked quinoa with banana, oat flour, and a bit of maple syrup. Fold in some chocolate chips or dried fruit before baking. These muffins are a nutrient-dense option lacking the empty calories often found in traditional breakfast pastries.

As the day progresses, quinoa proves to be just as dynamic and exciting in lunch applications. Quinoa salads are particularly excellent for meal prep since they store well in the fridge for several days. A classic Mediterranean quinoa salad can be your go-to. Combine cooked quinoa with cherry tomatoes, cucumbers, Kalamata olives, red onions, feta cheese, and fresh parsley. Dress it with olive oil, lemon juice, salt, and pepper. This salad is a vibrant, colorful mosaic packed with flavors and nutrients that can stand alone or complement a piece of grilled chicken or fish.

Seeking a warm, comfort-food alternative for lunch? Look no further than a quinoa vegetable stir-fry. Start with a base of sautéed garlic and onions; add your choice of vegetables like bell peppers, broccoli, and snap peas. Toss in cooked quinoa and a splash of soy sauce, and you've got yourself a filling, nutritious meal. The quinoa absorbs the flavors beautifully, creating a richly textured dish that's both satisfying and healthy.

Now, let's transition to dinner, where quinoa really shines as a versatile staple. One of the beauties of quinoa is that it can easily replace less nutritious options like white rice or pasta. For instance, a bowl of quinoa risotto with mushrooms can be both comforting and rich in umami flavors without the excess carbs found in traditional risotto. Use vegetable broth and a mix of wild mushrooms; finish with a drizzle of truffle oil if you're feeling fancy.

Another delicious dinner option is quinoa-stuffed bell peppers. These colorful creations are not just visually appealing but also packed with nutrients. Prepare the stuffing by mixing quinoa with black beans, corn, diced tomatoes, and spices like cumin and smoked paprika. Fill halved bell peppers with this mixture and bake until the peppers are tender. Top with avocado slices or even a sprinkle of shredded cheese for an added layer of taste.

To spice things up, quinoa can also be used as the base for a nutrient-rich, hearty soup. Quinoa soup, featuring an array of vegetables and beans, can be a one-pot wonder. Start by sautéing onions, garlic, and carrots; add broth, quinoa, and beans of your choice (like kidney or cannellini). Season with herbs such as thyme and bay leaves. The result is a comforting yet light dish that's perfect for any evening.

For those with a penchant for global cuisines, quinoa is versatile enough to fit into almost any culinary tradition. Take a Middle Eastern-inspired quinoa tabbouleh, for example. This dish swaps traditional bulgur wheat for quinoa, adding a complete protein element. Mix cooked quinoa with plenty of chopped parsley, mint, tomatoes, and diced cucumbers. Dress it with olive oil and lemon juice for a zesty, refreshing salad that could easily be the star of your dinner table.

And let's not forget about dessert. Yes, quinoa can enter the dessert realm. Quinoa pudding, similar to rice pudding, can be a nutritious way to end your day. Cook quinoa in coconut milk, adding sweeteners like maple syrup or agave nectar. Stir in some vanilla extract and top with fresh mango pieces or a dash of cinnamon. This dessert manages to feel indulgent while still being aligned with your health goals.

The adaptability of quinoa extends beyond fixed recipes. Don't hesitate to incorporate it into your favorite dishes. Swap it into stews, blend it into smoothie bowls, or even use it as a crispy coating for baked fish. The options are practically limitless, and the health benefits are robust. By integrating quinoa into breakfast, lunch, and dinner, you're making a commitment to a more nutrient-dense, balanced diet.

In summary, **Quinoa for Breakfast, Lunch, and Dinner** exemplifies how one superfood can fit seamlessly into every mealtime, offering a combination of convenience, taste, and superior nutrition. Whether you're starting your day with a quinoa-based meal, having it in a vibrant lunchtime salad, or ending with a hearty dinner dish, this versatile superfood makes it easy to meet your health goals without compromising on flavor or creativity. Embrace quinoa, and watch as it transforms your eating habits and contributes notably to your overall well-being.

brown rice: a staple for longevity

Brown rice stands out as a cornerstone of whole grains, offering a wealth of health benefits that contribute to a longer, more vibrant life. Unlike its refined counterpart, brown rice retains its nutrient-rich bran and germ layers, making it a powerhouse of fiber, vitamins, and minerals. This whole grain is particularly rich in magnesium, which plays a crucial role in numerous bodily functions, including energy production and DNA synthesis. Brown rice also boasts a low glycemic index, supporting stable blood sugar levels and reducing the risk of chronic conditions like diabetes and heart disease. Incorporating brown rice into your diet can be as simple as replacing white rice in your favorite dishes, thereby enhancing their nutritional profile without sacrificing flavor. From stir-fries and salads to hearty bowls and even desserts, brown rice proves to be a versatile superfood that's easy to enjoy daily.

Brown Rice Meal Ideas Brown rice is a dependable whole grain that's rich in fiber, antioxidants, and essential vitamins and minerals. Including it in your diet can significantly enhance your well-being. One of the great things about brown rice is its versatility—it can be incorporated into a plethora of dishes, from hearty mains to delectable desserts.

Let's start with the basics: a simple brown rice bowl. Cooked brown rice serves as an excellent base to which you can add a variety of toppings. Think sautéed vegetables like bell peppers, zucchini, and spinach. Add a protein source such as grilled tofu or baked chicken breast, and you've got a balanced and nutritious meal. Top it off with a drizzle of tahini or a sprinkle of sesame seeds for added flavor and nutrients.

Another fantastic option is a brown rice salad. Cook your brown rice and let it cool. Then mix it with chopped cucumbers, cherry tomatoes, red onions, and fresh herbs like parsley or cilantro. Dress it with olive oil and lemon juice; it's a light yet nourishing dish perfect for lunch or a side.

If you're looking for something more robust, consider making a brown rice stir-fry. Using a large skillet, heat some coconut oil and add minced garlic and ginger. After a minute or two, toss in your choice of vegetables such as broccoli, carrots, and snap peas. Once they start to soften, add your cooked brown rice and a splash of soy sauce. Stir it all together until well-mixed and heated through. For extra protein, include scrambled eggs or tofu cubes. This method allows you to use whatever vegetables you have on hand, reducing food waste while making a tasty, nutrient-dense meal.

For breakfast lovers, brown rice can also shine in the morning. Try a brown rice porridge by cooking the rice with almond milk until it reaches a creamy consistency. Sweeten it naturally with a bit of honey or maple syrup, and sprinkle some cinnamon and fresh fruit like blueberries or sliced bananas on top. It's a warming, filling breakfast option that provides sustained energy throughout the morning.

Moving onto global cuisine, brown rice works wonderfully in dishes like sushi and burritos. For sushi, use short-grain brown rice seasoned with rice vinegar. Lay a sheet of nori, spread the rice evenly, and add thinly sliced avocado, cucumber, or even grilled shrimp before rolling it up. This healthier twist on sushi offers the same delightful flavors but with the added benefits of whole grains.

For a Tex-Mex meal, make brown rice burritos. Cook the rice with some cumin and garlic, then layer it into a whole grain tortilla with black beans, corn, diced tomatoes, and a sprinkle of cheese. Add a dollop of guacamole or salsa, roll it up, and you have a wholesome, hand-held meal perfect for any time of day.

Soups and stews also benefit from the inclusion of brown rice. A personal favorite is a lentil and brown rice soup. In a large pot, sauté onions, garlic, and carrots in olive oil. Add lentils, a bay leaf, and some vegetable broth, and let it simmer. When the lentils are almost done, stir in your cooked brown rice. The result is a hearty, comforting soup that's packed with protein, fiber, and essential nutrients.

Brown rice also lends itself well to casseroles. Try a baked brown rice and vegetable casserole. In a baking dish, combine cooked brown rice with sautéed mushrooms, zucchini, and bell peppers. Add a mixture of beaten eggs and shredded cheese over the top, then bake until golden and set. This dish is not only delicious but also easy to make ahead and reheat for a quick, satisfying dinner.

Don't forget desserts! Yes, brown rice can even find its way into your dessert menu. Create a creamy rice pudding by simmering cooked brown rice with coconut milk, a bit of sweetener, and vanilla extract. Serve it warm or chilled, with a sprinkle of cinnamon or nutmeg. This dessert is both satisfying and nutritious, offering a healthier alternative to traditional sweets.

Brown rice can also be incorporated into more unique recipes like stuffed peppers. Hollow out bell peppers and stuff them with a mixture of brown rice, chopped vegetables, and spices. Bake until the peppers are tender—this makes for a colorful, nutrient-dense dish that's as appealing to the eyes as it is to the palate.

When you're pressed for time, a quick brown rice and beans dish can be a lifesaver. Heat up some canned black beans with spices like cumin and chili powder. Serve over a bed of brown rice, and garnish with sliced avocado, fresh lime juice, and chopped cilantro. This meal is both speedy and nutrient-packed, providing a good balance of protein, fiber, and healthy fats.

In summary, brown rice is a versatile and health-boosting ingredient that can be used in a wide variety of dishes. From simple rice bowls and salads to more complex casseroles and desserts, the possibilities are endless. By making brown rice a regular part of your diet, you will not only enjoy its rich, nutty flavor but also reap numerous health benefits that contribute to longevity and overall wellness.

Chapter 5:
Nuts and Seeds

Nuts and seeds are power-packed nuggets of nutrition, offering a myriad of health benefits that support both vitality and longevity. These tiny yet mighty foods are brimming with essential fatty acids, protein, fiber, vitamins, and minerals, making them indispensable in any health-conscious diet. Rich in heart-healthy fats, nuts like almonds can help reduce bad cholesterol levels, while seeds such as chia are known for their omega-3 fatty acids, which support brain health. Not only do they provide energy and satiety, but their antioxidant properties also help combat oxidative stress, potentially reducing the risk of chronic diseases. Incorporating a variety of nuts and seeds into your daily meals or snacks is a simple yet effective way to boost your overall well-being, providing sustained energy and a wealth of nutrients your body craves.

Chia Seeds: Tiny but Mighty

Chia seeds may be small in size, but they pack a powerful punch when it comes to nutrition and health benefits. These tiny seeds are rich in omega-3 fatty acids, which are essential for heart health and reducing inflammation. They also provide a significant amount of fiber, aiding in digestion and helping to maintain a feeling of fullness, which is great for weight management. Moreover, chia seeds are loaded with antioxidants and essential minerals like calcium, magnesium, and iron, supporting strong bones and overall vitality. Incorporating chia seeds into your diet is simple and versatile; you can sprinkle them into smoothies, mix them into yogurt, or use them as a base for nutrient-packed puddings. By adding these mighty seeds to your daily routine, you not only boost nutrient intake but also enhance your overall well-being.

Chia Seed Pudding and Beyond is a delightful, versatile way to enjoy one of nature's most nutrient-packed seeds. These tiny black or white seeds, originating from the Salvia hispanica plant, have been recognized for their health benefits for centuries. Modern science reveals that chia seeds are loaded with fiber, protein, omega-3 fatty acids, and various micronutrients. Moreover, they have the unique ability to absorb liquid, expanding up to ten times their weight, which makes them perfect for creating pudding-like textures without added thickeners.

Imagine starting your day with a chia seed pudding; it's not just a healthy choice but also a gastronomic experience. The basic recipe couldn't be simpler—mix chia seeds with your favorite plant-based milk, let it sit overnight, and voilà! By morning, you'll have a creamy, satisfying pudding ready to be topped with fruits, nuts, or even a drizzle of honey.

But chia seed pudding is just the beginning. You can elevate this basic recipe by incorporating a variety of superfoods. For instance, mixing in matcha powder can not only enhance the flavor but also provide a boost of antioxidants. Alternatively, adding a spoonful of acai or spirulina will introduce additional nutrients and vibrant colors to your dish.

Another exciting avenue to explore is using chia seeds in savory dishes. Imagine a chia seed and herb-infused dressing for your salads, or a chia seed and flax blend that you can sprinkle over roasted vegetables. The gelatinous quality of soaked chia seeds makes it an excellent binder for plant-based burgers or falafels, adding both texture and nutritional value.

One of the most overlooked benefits of chia seeds is their role in hydration. Because chia seeds absorb so much liquid, consuming them can help you stay hydrated longer—a crucial aspect, especially during strenuous activities or hot weather. A refreshing chia fresca, made by mixing chia seeds with water, lemon juice, and a touch of sweetener, is a fantastic, hydrating beverage that's easy to prepare and enjoy on the go.

Understanding the versatility of chia seeds opens up endless culinary possibilities. Picture this: chia seeds added to your morning smoothie, creating a thicker, more filling drink without altering the taste significantly. Or how about a chia seed jam where chia seeds absorb the fruit juices, eliminating the need for added sugars or pectin?

Chia seeds can also be a wonderful addition to your baking repertoire. They can replace eggs in vegan baking recipes—a simple mixture of one tablespoon of chia seeds to three tablespoons of water creates a chia 'egg'. This not only helps bind the ingredients together but also boosts the nutritional profile of your baked goods. Imagine chia-enhanced muffins, pancakes, or even energy bars.

Incorporating chia seeds into your diet also aligns with a more sustainable and health-conscious lifestyle. Chia plants require relatively little water to grow, making them an environmentally friendly crop. Plus, their long shelf life means you can buy them in bulk, reducing packaging waste and frequent trips to the store.

For those looking to integrate chia seeds more seamlessly into their diet, chia supplements are another viable option. Available in various forms like powders or capsules, these supplements offer an easy way to ensure you're getting your daily dose of this superfood without having to think too much about it. Of course, it is always best to consume chia seeds in their whole form to maximize fiber intake and enjoy the full sensory experience.

The health benefits of chia seeds go beyond just fiber and omega-3s. They're also rich in essential minerals like calcium, magnesium, and phosphorus, which are crucial for maintaining healthy bones and metabolic functions. In addition, the antioxidants in chia seeds help combat free radicals in the body, potentially lowering the risk of chronic diseases.

For fitness enthusiasts, chia seeds are a powerhouse of plant-based protein. Incorporating them into your post-workout snacks can promote muscle recovery and sustain energy levels. A chia protein smoothie bowl, for example, can be both a nutritious and tasty way to replenish after a strenuous workout.

Chia seed pudding and beyond offer more than just a delicious treat; they are an entry point into a more mindful, nutrient-rich lifestyle. By experimenting with different recipes and combinations, you can enjoy the numerous health benefits that chia seeds offer while adding variety and excitement to your meals.

Let's explore some fun and practical ways to make the most out of chia seeds. How about a chia fruit parfait, layering chia pudding with Greek yogurt and fresh berries? This can serve as an exquisite breakfast or a refreshing evening snack. The possibilities are truly endless and limited only by your culinary creativity.

Chia seeds are also excellent for anyone following a gluten-free or grain-free diet. They can be used to create bread or crackers, providing that much-needed crunch without the gluten. For instance, a simple mixture of chia seeds, water, and seasoning baked finely can yield crispy, nutritious crackers perfect for snacking or as a base for appetizers.

In sum, the humble chia seed's potential extends far beyond the popular pudding. From smoothies and baking to savory dishes and hydration solutions, chia seeds can be a versatile and invaluable addition to your diet. Embrace the possibilities and start experimenting with chia seeds in various forms—your body will thank you.

Almonds: A Crunchy Source of Energy

Almonds are a powerhouse of nutrition, making them an excellent choice for those looking to boost their energy levels naturally. Packed with healthy fats, protein, and fiber, almonds provide a satisfying crunch while delivering sustained energy throughout the day. They're rich in vitamins and minerals such as vitamin E, magnesium, and calcium, all of which contribute to overall well-being. Whether you're tossing them into a salad, blending them into a smoothie, or simply enjoying a handful as a snack, almonds offer versatile and tasty ways to enhance your diet. Their nutrient profile supports cardiovascular health, aids in weight management, and promotes healthy skin, making them a crucial addition to any health-conscious individual's pantry.

Snacking Smart with Almond Recipes involves more than just grabbing a handful of these nutrient-packed nuts; it's about integrating them creatively into your daily routine. Almonds are a powerhouse of essential nutrients like vitamin E, magnesium, and healthy fats that contribute significantly to overall health and longevity. Incorporating almonds in different snack recipes not only adds a delightful crunch but also helps in keeping your energy levels stable throughout the day. Whether you're looking for a quick bite between meals or a nutritious addition to your salads, we have a variety of almond-based recipes to get you started.

When you're on the go and need a quick snack, consider making almond energy bites. These tiny yet mighty morsels are packed with nutrients and can be prepared in advance, making them an ideal choice for busy days. Simply blend almonds with dates, a touch of honey, and perhaps a sprinkle of cacao for a chocolatey kick. Roll the mixture into small balls and store them in the fridge. You'll have an energizing, healthy snack ready whenever you need it.

For those who appreciate a more savory option, almond-crusted avocado is a must-try. This innovative recipe combines the creamy richness of avocados with the crunchy texture of crushed almonds. Slice your avocado into wedges, dip them in beaten egg, then coat them generously with finely chopped almonds. Bake in a preheated oven until golden brown. Not only is this snack delicious, but it's also incredibly satisfying and rich in healthy fats and fiber.

If you're a fan of smoothies, adding almond butter to your blend can take your drink to the next level. Almond butter adds a creamy texture and a nutty flavor that pairs well with a variety of fruits and vegetables. Blend a tablespoon of almond butter with spinach, a banana, a handful of berries, and some almond milk for a smoothie that's not only tasty but also packed with vitamins, minerals, and antioxidants. It's a fantastic way to start your day or refuel after a workout.

Another delightful way to enjoy almonds is by preparing almond granola bars. These bars are perfect for a mid-morning snack or a light afternoon bite. Mix rolled oats, chopped almonds, dried fruit, and a bit of honey or maple syrup. Press the mixture into a baking dish and bake until golden. Once cooled, cut into bars and store in an airtight container. These bars are not only delicious but also help in sustaining your energy levels, thanks to the complex carbs and healthy fats.

For a gourmet touch to your snacks, try making almond-stuffed dates. This recipe is as simple as it gets but offers a delectable combination of flavors and textures. Remove the pits from dates and stuff each one with a whole almond. You can take it a step further by adding a small dollop of almond butter inside each date before placing the almond. These make for a sweet, satisfying snack that's perfect for curbing those mid-afternoon sugar cravings without the added guilt of processed sweets.

If you prefer your snacks with a bit of spice, roasted almonds with a hint of chili and lime can be your go-to. Toss raw almonds with a splash of lime juice, chili powder, and a pinch of salt. Spread them out on a baking sheet and roast until they're just right. The combination of heat from the chili and the tangy lime flavor creates an addictive snack that's hard to resist. Plus, roasting them gives the almonds a deeper flavor and a delicious crunch.

Incorporating almonds into your diet doesn't always have to be about snacks; they can also be a great addition to your salads. Toasted almonds add a delightful crunch and a burst of flavor to any green salad. Just toss a handful of sliced almonds into a dry skillet over medium heat and stir them occasionally until they become golden brown and fragrant. Sprinkle them over your favorite salad mix—whether it's a combination of leafy greens, fruits, and a light vinaigrette, or a hearty bowl of grains and veggies.

For those who enjoy baking, almond flour can be a fantastic gluten-free alternative to traditional wheat flour. It adds a moist, rich texture to baked goods while providing the health benefits associated with almonds. Try making almond flour muffins or cookies as part of your snacking routine. These treats will not only satisfy your sweet tooth but also deliver a dose of protein, healthy fats, and fiber.

Using almonds in homemade trail mix is another excellent way to enjoy their benefits. Combine almonds with other nuts, dried fruits, and some dark chocolate chunks for a mix that's both nutritious and delicious. This trail mix can be portioned into small containers or zip-lock bags, making it an easy grab-and-go option for hiking trips, office snacks, or any time you need a quick, nutritious pick-me-up.

For a snack that feels a bit more indulgent, consider making chocolate-covered almonds. Melt some dark chocolate, which itself is a superfood, and dip each almond until it's well-coated. Let them cool on a sheet of parchment paper until the chocolate hardens. These make for an excellent treat that combines the antioxidants from the dark chocolate with the various health benefits of almonds.

Finally, one of the simplest ways to enjoy almonds is by making your own almond milk. It's surprisingly easy to do and offers a nutritious alternative to cow's milk. Soak a cup of raw almonds overnight, then drain and rinse them. Blend the almonds with four cups of water until smooth, then strain the mixture through a nut milk bag or a fine-mesh sieve lined with cheesecloth. The result is a creamy, delicious almond milk that you can use in smoothies, coffee, or just drink on its own. Store it in the fridge and enjoy it over the next few days.

Snacking Smart with Almond Recipes is all about making the most of this versatile, nutritious nut. Whether you're in the mood for something sweet, savory, or somewhere in between, there's an almond recipe that can satisfy your cravings while contributing to your overall health and longevity. In the following sections, we'll explore more ways to incorporate nutrient-dense superfoods into your diet, empowering you to lead a healthier, more vibrant life.

Chapter 6:
Legumes

Legumes stand as one of the most underrated yet transformative food groups you can introduce to your diet for enhanced health and longevity. Packed with protein, fiber, and essential vitamins and minerals, legumes such as lentils, chickpeas, and beans offer immense versatility and nutrient density. They boast a low glycemic index, making them an excellent choice for sustained energy levels and blood sugar management. Their rich fiber content not only aids digestion but also supports heart health by helping to lower bad cholesterol. Additionally, legumes are environmentally friendly, requiring fewer resources to grow compared to animal-based proteins. By integrating legumes into meals like soups, salads, or stews, you can effortlessly enrich your diet and contribute to a sustainable future.

Lentils: The Versatile Superfood

Among the treasures in the legume family, lentils stand out for their remarkable versatility and nutritional profile. These tiny, lens-shaped pulses are packed with protein, fiber, and essential vitamins and minerals such as folate, iron, and magnesium. Whether you incorporate them into soups, stews, salads, or even as a meat substitute in various dishes, lentils offer a hearty and satisfying way to boost your diet. Their quick cooking time and ability to absorb flavors make them a favorite in numerous culinary traditions around the world, ensuring you can enjoy both their nutrient density and delightful taste with ease. Embrace lentils in your daily meals and experience not only their health benefits but also the rich, diverse textures and flavors they bring to your table.

Lentil Soups and Stews provide a delicious and effective way to harness the nutritional power of lentils. Lentils, a staple in many global cuisines, are renowned for their high protein, fiber, and a multitude of essential vitamins and minerals. Lentils come in several varieties such as green, brown, red, and black, each bringing its own unique texture and flavor to a dish. Whether you're aiming for a hearty and filling meal or a lighter, brothy soup, lentil-based recipes can suit any preference or dietary need.

When it comes to preparing **Lentil Soups and Stews**, versatility is key. You can mix lentils with a variety of vegetables, spices, and even meats, although they shine just as brightly in vegetarian and vegan preparations. One popular approach is to start with a mirepoix— a combination of onions, carrots, and celery—sautéed in a bit of olive oil. This creates a flavorful foundation that complements the earthy taste of the lentils. From there, you can add your lentils, broth or water, and let everything simmer until the lentils are tender.

The nutritional profile of **Lentil Soups and Stews** is impressive. Lentils are rich in protein, making them an excellent meat substitute, particularly in vegetarian or vegan diets. They're also packed with essential nutrients such as folate, iron, and magnesium. The fiber content of lentils can't be overstated; it aids in digestion and helps maintain stable blood sugar levels, making these soups and stews not just comforting, but also beneficial for long-term health.

Seasoning your **Lentil Soups and Stews** is where creativity comes into play. Options are endless, from the warming spices of a curry lentil soup to the smoky, robust flavors of a lentil and sausage stew. Using fresh herbs like cilantro or parsley can brighten the dish, while a squeeze of lemon juice or a splash of apple cider vinegar can add a tangy finish. A popular spice combination includes cumin, coriander, and turmeric, which not only adds flavor but also infuses the stew with additional anti-inflammatory properties.

In addition to delicious flavor, the ease of preparing **Lentil Soups and Stews** makes them a perfect addition to any meal plan. Lentils don't require soaking, drastically reducing prep time. This means you can often go from ingredients to a finished dish in under an hour. For busy individuals, recipes that involve minimal hands-on time but yield nutritious, satisfying results are invaluable. Simply put, it's hard to beat a pot of lentil soup simmering on the stove after a long day.

Incorporating **Lentil Soups and Stews** into your diet is made even easier with one-pot recipes. These minimize cleanup and simplify the cooking process. For example, a lentil and vegetable stew can include a diverse mix of whatever vegetables you have on hand—from potatoes and tomatoes to kale and spinach. All ingredients cook together, allowing their flavors to meld beautifully. Such recipes are excellent for meal prep, as the flavors often deepen and improve after a day or two in the refrigerator.

For those seeking to boost their intake of plant-based proteins, **Lentil Soups and Stews** offer a scientific and nutritious solution. Studies have shown that regularly consuming legumes like lentils can contribute to heart health, reduce cholesterol levels, and even support weight management. Undoubtedly, lentils are a key player in the quest for longevity and well-being. Their inclusion in soups and stews makes them not only accessible but also enjoyable for people of all ages.

Lentil soup recipes also offer cultural diversity, embracing flavors from around the world. Middle Eastern lentil soups, for instance, often incorporate cumin, coriander, and fresh lemon juice, creating a flavorful, aromatic dish. Indian lentil soups, or dals, are typically enriched with a blend of spices like turmeric, cumin, and garam masala, resulting in a rich and complex flavor profile. These global culinary traditions highlight the lentil's adaptability and endless possibilities.

Furthermore, **Lentil Soups and Stews** can be customized to seasonal availability. In the winter months, they can feature root vegetables and hearty greens, creating a robust and warming dish. Conversely, in warmer seasons, they can be made with lighter broths and fresh summer vegetables. This seasonal adaptability not only keeps meals interesting but also ensures you're taking advantage of the freshest and most nutrient-dense ingredients available.

For an added nutritional boost, consider incorporating other superfoods into your **Lentil Soups and Stews**. Leafy greens like kale and spinach can enhance the nutritional profile, providing additional vitamins and minerals. Incorporating whole grains like quinoa or barley can further enrich the stew, adding both texture and an extra dose of fiber. Additionally, supplementing with nuts and seeds, such as a sprinkle of chia seeds, can introduce healthy fats and additional protein, making the meal even more balanced and fulfilling.

In summary, **Lentil Soups and Stews** are not only delicious but also an incredible vehicle for superfood nutrition. They're versatile, easy to prepare, and customizable to suit different tastes and dietary preferences. Their rich nutritional profile can significantly contribute to overall health and longevity, aligning perfectly with the goals of embracing a superfood-rich diet. So next time you're looking for a comforting, nutritious meal, remember that a pot of lentil soup or stew can be your go-to option, combining simplicity with the profound benefits of superfoods.

Chickpeas: More Than Just Hummus

When you think of chickpeas, hummus might be the first thing that comes to mind, but this versatile legume has so much more to offer. Packed with protein, fiber, vitamins, and minerals, chickpeas can elevate a variety of dishes, from salads and soups to stews and even baked goods. These nutrient-dense gems are not only a staple in Mediterranean and Middle Eastern cuisines but also an excellent meat substitute in vegetarian and vegan diets. They're great for enhancing digestive health, supporting weight management, and helping to maintain stable blood sugar levels. Chickpeas add both texture and nutrition to your meals, ensuring that you're not just eating well but thriving. They make it easier than ever to incorporate superfoods into your everyday routine, turning simple meals into health-boosting endeavors. So, next time you're thinking about what to cook, remember that chickpeas can be your go-to ingredient for a nutritious and delicious dish beyond just hummus.

Creative Chickpea Dishes Chickpeas, also known as garbanzo beans, are more than just the core ingredient for hummus. They are versatile, nutrient-rich legumes that lend themselves to a myriad of culinary creations. In this section, we'll explore inventive ways to incorporate chickpeas into your meals, extending far beyond traditional uses. Chickpeas are rich in protein, fiber, vitamins, and minerals, making them a superfood that can significantly contribute to a balanced, health-enhancing diet.

One of the simplest and most delicious ways to enjoy chickpeas is by roasting them. Roasted chickpeas make for a crunchy, satisfying snack that's easy to prepare and perfect for on-the-go snacking. Simply toss drained and rinsed chickpeas in olive oil with your favorite spices—try paprika, cumin, and a pinch of sea salt—then spread them out on a baking sheet and roast at 400°F for about 20-30 minutes. You'll know they're done when they're golden brown and crispy. Not only are roasted chickpeas a tasty snack, but they can also be used as a crunchy topping for salads and soups.

Why not elevate your breakfast game by adding chickpeas to your morning routine? A chickpea scramble is a fantastic alternative to the traditional egg scramble, especially for those following a plant-based diet. Start by heating some olive oil in a skillet and sautéing diced onions, bell peppers, and tomatoes. Add in chickpeas that have been lightly mashed with a fork to create a scrambled texture. Season with turmeric, salt, and pepper. Cook until everything is heated through and combined. Serve with whole-grain toast or wrapped in a whole-wheat tortilla for a nutritious start to your day.

Chickpeas also shine in soups and stews, providing a hearty addition that boosts the nutritional value of your meal. Consider making a Moroccan-inspired chickpea stew. Begin by sautéing onions, garlic, and ginger in a large pot. Add in spices like cumin, coriander, cinnamon, and a bit of cayenne pepper. Throw in chopped tomatoes, vegetable broth, and chickpeas. Let the stew simmer until the flavors meld together, and finish with a handful of fresh spinach or kale. This dish is not only packed with flavor but also offers a warm, comforting meal rich in essential nutrients.

For those who love Mediterranean flavors, a chickpea salad is a refreshing and nutrient-dense option. Combine cooked chickpeas with an array of colorful vegetables such as cherry tomatoes, cucumbers, red onions, and bell peppers. Toss in some Kalamata olives and feta cheese for an extra burst of flavor. Dress the salad with a simple vinaigrette made from olive oil, lemon juice, minced garlic, and oregano. This salad can be served as a main dish or a side, providing a fresh, satisfying experience with every bite.

Even desserts can benefit from the addition of chickpeas. Chickpea blondies are a healthier twist on the traditional dessert. Blend chickpeas with almond butter, maple syrup, vanilla extract, a pinch of salt, and a leavening agent like baking powder until smooth. Fold in some dark chocolate chips and spread the mixture into a baking dish. Bake at 350°F for about 20-25 minutes until the blondies are set. The result is a dessert that's rich in protein and fiber, making it a treat you can enjoy without the guilt.

Another innovative dish is chickpea pasta, which has gained popularity as a gluten-free alternative to traditional pasta. Made from chickpea flour, this pasta is higher in protein and fiber than its wheat counterpart. You can prepare it like any other pasta by boiling it until al dente, then tossing it with your favorite sauce. For a simple yet delectable meal, try chickpea pasta with a tomato basil sauce. Sauté garlic in olive oil, add canned crushed tomatoes, season with salt, pepper, and fresh basil, and combine with cooked chickpea pasta. Top with a sprinkle of nutritional yeast or Parmesan cheese, depending on your dietary preferences.

If you're a fan of burgers but looking for a plant-based option, chickpea patties are an excellent choice. To make these, blend chickpeas with garlic, onions, parsley, spices like cumin and coriander, and a binder such as breadcrumbs or oat flour. Shape the mixture into patties and pan-fry them in a bit of oil until golden brown on both sides. Serve them on whole-grain buns with your favorite toppings. These chickpea patties are not only delicious but also packed with protein and fiber, making them a nutritious and satisfying meal.

Chickpeas are also incredibly versatile in curries, absorbing the flavors of the various spices used. A classic chickpea curry can be made by cooking onions, garlic, and ginger until fragrant, then adding a mix of spices like garam masala, turmeric, and cumin. Throw in tomatoes and coconut milk for a creamy base, followed by the chickpeas. Simmer until the chickpeas are tender and the flavors have melded together. Serve over brown rice or quinoa for a complete and balanced meal.

For a fusion of flavors, try chickpea tacos. These can be as simple or elaborate as you like. Start by marinating chickpeas in a mix of lime juice, chili powder, cumin, and salt. Sauté the marinated chickpeas in a skillet until heated through and slightly crispy. Serve them in corn tortillas with toppings like shredded cabbage, sliced avocado, fresh cilantro, and a drizzle of tahini sauce. Chickpea tacos are a delightful way to add more legumes to your diet while enjoying a burst of different flavors and textures.

Chickpeas can even make their way into your beverages. Yes, you read that right! Aquafaba, the liquid found in a can of chickpeas, is a magical ingredient that can be used to create an array of recipes, including cocktails and mocktails. Whip aquafaba like you would egg whites to add a frothy texture to drinks, or use it as a vegan substitute in recipes requiring meringue.

Lastly, don't underestimate the power of a classic hummus. While traditional hummus is well-known, you can get creative by adding different flavors. Think roasted red pepper, sun-dried tomato, or even beetroot for a vibrant twist. These variations not only add a splash of color to your dish but also contribute additional nutrients and antioxidants. Serve hummus as a dip with fresh vegetables, spread it on sandwiches, or use it as a base for grain bowls.

In conclusion, chickpeas are an incredibly versatile superfood that can be adapted to all kinds of dishes, from snacks to main courses to desserts. Their high protein and fiber content, along with their adaptability to various flavors and cuisines, make them a valuable addition to any diet. Whether you're looking to enhance your health, explore new recipes, or simply enjoy delicious food, chickpeas offer endless possibilities. So don't limit yourself to just hummus—bring the humble chickpea into the spotlight and let it transform your meals.

Chapter 7:
Fermented Foods

Fermented foods are a treasure trove of beneficial probiotics that can drastically improve gut health and overall well-being. Incorporating options like kombucha, kefir, and other cultured delights into your diet can boost your digestive system and enhance nutrient absorption, thanks to the presence of good bacteria and vital nutrients. These foods work continuously to balance your gut's microflora, making digestion smoother and lowering inflammation. With options ranging from fermented vegetables to cultured dairy, fermented foods are versatile and can easily be included in daily meals. By embracing these flavorful and health-promoting foods, you're giving your body a natural tool to maintain its health and longevity.

kombucha: the probiotic power drink

In the realm of fermented foods, kombucha stands out as a probiotic powerhouse with a rich history and a myriad of health benefits. Made from sweetened tea fermented by a symbiotic culture of bacteria and yeast (SCOBY), kombucha is renowned for its gut-friendly properties. Incorporating this effervescent drink into your diet can support digestion, boost your immune system, and provide a natural source of energy. The tangy, slightly vinegary flavor has captivated health enthusiasts worldwide, who appreciate its unique taste and nutritional profile. To get the most out of kombucha, consider starting with small amounts and gradually increasing your intake, ensuring your gut has time to adjust to this potent elixir.

Brewing Kombucha at Home is not just a culinary adventure; it's an investment in your health and longevity. Kombucha is a fermented tea rich in probiotics, enzymes, and organic acids that work in harmony to improve digestion, boost the immune system, and even enhance mental clarity. The beauty of brewing kombucha at home lies in its accessibility and customization, allowing you to incorporate various superfoods to maximize its health benefits.

To start, you'll need a few essential ingredients and equipment: a quality SCOBY (Symbiotic Culture of Bacteria and Yeast), black or green tea, cane sugar, purified water, and a fermentation vessel, typically a glass jar. The SCOBY is the heart and soul of your kombucha, driving the fermentation process and enriching the tea with beneficial probiotics.

Step-by-Step Guide to Brewing Kombucha

1. Preparing the Sweet Tea Base: Begin by boiling 1 gallon of purified water. Once boiled, add 4-5 tea bags of black or green tea and let them steep for about 10-15 minutes. Remove the tea bags and stir in 1 cup of cane sugar until fully dissolved. Allow the sweetened tea to cool to room temperature. This step is crucial, as adding the SCOBY to hot tea can harm or kill the beneficial bacteria and yeast.

2. Introducing the SCOBY: Transfer the cooled sweet tea into your fermentation vessel. Carefully place the SCOBY in the tea, making sure it floats on the surface. Add 1-2 cups of already brewed kombucha (this can be store-bought or from a previous batch) to acidify the mixture and jumpstart the fermentation process.

The fermentation vessel should be covered with a breathable cloth or paper towel secured with a rubber band. This allows the kombucha to breathe while keeping out contaminants like dust and insects. Place the jar in a warm, dark place with a temperature range of 68-85°F (20-29°C). Avoid direct sunlight, as too much light can interfere with the fermentation.

During the first few days, you'll notice bubbles forming and the SCOBY might rise, sink, or float sideways in the tea, all of which are normal behaviors. A new, thinner SCOBY typically starts forming on the surface of the tea. Allow the mixture to ferment for 7 to 10 days, tasting it periodically from day 7 onwards. The longer the kombucha ferments, the less sweet and more tart it becomes.

3. Bottling and Flavoring: When your kombucha reaches the desired balance of sweetness and tartness, it's time for the second fermentation (optional but recommended for added flavor and carbonation). Remove the SCOBY and 1-2 cups of the kombucha liquid to use as a starter for your next batch. Pour the remaining kombucha into airtight bottles, leaving a little room at the top for flavor additions and carbonation.

This is where you can get creative with superfoods. Add fresh ginger slices, berries, herbs like mint or basil, or even superfood powders like spirulina or turmeric. Seal the bottles tightly and allow them to ferment at room temperature for an additional 3 to 7 days. This secondary fermentation period enhances the flavors and creates natural carbonation.

After the second fermentation, refrigerate the bottles. Cold storage slows down the fermentation process, giving you a refreshing, fizzy drink. Always open your bottles carefully, as the pressure can build up over time. Enjoy your homemade kombucha as a delicious, probiotic-rich alternative to sugary drinks and sodas.

Kombucha offers endless possibilities for customization. Experimenting with different types of tea, sugars, and flavorings can result in unique and delightful brews. Green tea kombucha typically has a more delicate flavor, while black tea kombucha tends to be bolder and richer. You can also mix teas for a balanced profile.

Quality control is critical. Always use purified water to avoid introducing chlorine or other contaminants that can hinder fermentation. Cleanliness is paramount; sanitize your equipment to prevent unwanted bacteria or mold from contaminating your brew. If you notice off-putting smells or visible mold on your SCOBY, discard the batch and start anew.

Health Benefits and Cautions

The health benefits of kombucha are numerous, thanks to its probiotic content. Probiotics aid digestion by replenishing the gut flora and supporting the immune system. Additionally, the organic acids produced during fermentation, such as acetic, lactic, and gluconic acids, can help detoxify the body, improve liver function, and even boost your mood by enhancing gut-brain communication.

However, moderation is key. Due to its acidity and potential alcohol content (typically 0.5-1%), it's best to consume kombucha in moderation, about 4-8 ounces a day. Overconsumption can lead to digestive discomfort or exacerbate pre-existing conditions like acid reflux.

When brewing kombucha at home, it's important to be mindful of safety. Improper fermentation or contamination can lead to harmful bacteria growth. Always be vigilant about cleanliness and monitor your kombucha for any signs of spoilage. If in doubt, it is safer to discard a questionable batch than to risk potential health hazards.

Brewing kombucha is an enjoyable and rewarding process that brings both immediate and long-term health benefits. With each batch, you invest in your well-being and open doors to creative, nutritious possibilities. By integrating this probiotic powerhouse into your diet, you take a significant step toward longevity and vitality, aligning beautifully with the holistic goals of incorporating superfoods into your daily life.

Kefir: Cultured Dairy for Gut Health

Kefir, a tangy and effervescent cultured dairy product, stands out in the realm of fermented foods for its remarkable contribution to gut health. Loaded with probiotics, kefir enhances digestion and supports a balanced microbiome, making it a staple for those seeking improved gastrointestinal well-being. More than just a probiotic powerhouse, kefir also boasts an impressive nutrient profile, rich in vitamins, minerals, and proteins that can help fortify the immune system. Incorporating kefir into your diet can be as simple as enjoying a glass on its own, blending it into smoothies, or using it as a base for salad dressings to imbue your meals with both flavor and health benefits. By making kefir a regular part of your dietary routine, you'll not only nourish your gut but also support overall vitality and longevity.

Incorporating Kefir into Your Meals is an excellent way to add both flavor and potent health benefits to your diet. Kefir, a cultured dairy product, is celebrated for its probiotic content which supports gut health. These live microorganisms are integral in maintaining a balanced intestinal flora, which can improve digestion, boost your immune system, and even enhance mental well-being.

Starting your morning with kefir can be a powerful routine. Consider swapping your usual yogurt or milk for kefir in breakfast smoothies. Mix one cup of kefir with some frozen berries, a banana, and a handful of spinach for a nutrient-packed start to the day. The tangy flavor of kefir blends seamlessly with the sweetness of fruit, creating a delicious and nutritious smoothie that even picky eaters might enjoy.

For a more traditional approach, pour kefir over a bowl of your favorite granola. The creamy texture of kefir complements the crunchiness of granola, and this combination creates a perfect balance of proteins, fibers, and healthy fats. Add in a drizzle of honey and a sprinkle of chia seeds to elevate the nutritional profile even further. From here, you can build and customize—adding nuts, seeds, or fruits to your taste.

Incorporating kefir into lunch meals can also be highly beneficial. Use kefir as the base for salad dressings. Replace buttermilk or mayonnaise in recipes with kefir to achieve that desired creamy consistency while keeping the calories in check. A tangy kefir-based dressing with lemon juice, olive oil, garlic, and dill can be both refreshing and satisfying, turning a simple salad into a delightful and nourishing meal.

Kefir's adaptability doesn't end with dressings. It's also an excellent ingredient in marinades for meat and fish. The acidity in kefir helps to tenderize meat, making it especially useful for tougher cuts. Marinate chicken breasts or fish fillets in a mixture of kefir, minced garlic, lemon zest, and herbs for a few hours before grilling or baking. This will not only enhance the flavor but also infuse the protein with beneficial probiotics.

As you move towards your evening meals, think about incorporating kefir into soups and stews. Adding kefir to your soup just before serving can enrich the flavor and add a creamier texture without the heaviness of cream. A dollop of kefir in a bowl of chilled gazpacho or a steaming cup of creamy mushroom soup can elevate your dining experience while boosting your meal's probiotic content.

For those who enjoy baking, kefir can be a secret weapon. Substitute kefir for milk or buttermilk in pancake, waffle, and muffin recipes. Its acidity reacts with baking soda to give a light and fluffy texture to baked goods. Picture a stack of blueberry kefir pancakes on a leisurely Sunday morning, topped with fresh fruit and a swirl of maple syrup.

If you're looking for snack ideas, kefir can be equally versatile. Prepare a simple kefir dip by mixing it with finely chopped cucumbers, garlic, dill, and a pinch of salt. This refreshing dip pairs wonderfully with sliced vegetables, whole grain crackers, or pita bread for a wholesome yet gratifying snack.

Incorporating kefir into your desserts offers a delightful and nutritious twist. Try making kefir-based parfaits by layering it with berries, nuts, and a hint of natural sweetener. The tang of kefir pairs well with the sweetness of fruits, creating a balanced and satisfying dessert. For a more indulgent yet healthy treat, kefir can be used in cheesecake recipes to replace the heavy cream cheese, giving the dessert a lighter texture without compromising on flavor.

One aspect that often goes unnoticed is how easily kefir integrates into savory dishes beyond marinades and dressings. Consider incorporating kefir in dishes like mashed potatoes or creamy pasta sauces. Replace some or all of the butter and cream with kefir to cut down on unhealthy fats while adding a subtle tang and a dose of probiotics to your meal.

For a quick and nutritious afternoon pick-me-up, try a kefir-based smoothie bowl. Blend kefir with your favorite fruits, pour it into a bowl, and layer it with toppings such as granola, seeds, nuts, and fresh berries. This not only makes for an Instagram-worthy snack but also provides a balanced mix of protein, fiber, and vitamins that can help curb afternoon cravings and sustain your energy levels until dinner.

Children can also benefit from the inclusion of kefir in their diets, albeit with a careful approach to flavors. You can introduce them to kefir without them even noticing it by incorporating it into popsicles. Blend kefir with fruit and a bit of natural sweetener, then freeze in molds. These homemade kefir popsicles are a fantastic way to get children to enjoy the benefits of probiotics while also treating them to a delicious, healthy snack.

Another creative way to use kefir is in savory pancakes or fritters. Mix kefir into the batter for zucchini fritters or even savory pancakes with herbs and spices. These can make a wonderful side dish or even a main dish when paired with a fresh salad. The kefir adds moisture and a unique flavor profile that stands out without overwhelming the other ingredients.

During the warmer months, chilled soups or cold kefir beverages are particularly refreshing. A traditional Eastern European beverage called kefir water can be made by blending kefir with chilled water, herbs, and a squeeze of lemon juice. It's a hydrating and cooling drink that offers a delightful alternative to more calorie-laden options.

Don't forget about kefir as a component in dressings and sauces for sandwiches and wraps. Its tangy flavor can balance richer fillings, whether you're assembling a veggie-stuffed wrap or a grilled chicken sandwich. A simple kefir sauce with lemon, dill, and cucumbers can make a notable difference in taste and nutrient content.

The beauty of kefir is its versatility. Whether you're aiming to boost the probiotic content of your meals, enhance the nutritional density of your food, or simply enjoy a delicious and refreshing ingredient, kefir offers countless opportunities. This means that with a little creativity, there are endless ways to incorporate kefir into your everyday meals, making it easier to stick to a nutritious diet without feeling limited or bored.

To wrap things up, kefir isn't just a health trend—it's a staple that can adapt to almost any meal, offering numerous health benefits along the way. From breakfast smoothies to dinner marinades and everything in between, incorporating kefir into your meals can be both a delicious and smart way to ensure you're nurturing your body with the nutrition it needs for longevity and overall well-being.

Chapter 8:
Healthy Oils

Incorporating healthy oils into your diet is a simple yet highly effective way to enhance overall well-being and longevity. Olive oil, often referred to as "liquid gold," is celebrated for its heart-healthy monounsaturated fats and robust antioxidant profile, making it an essential staple in any superfood-centric kitchen. Coconut oil, another versatile oil, boasts medium-chain triglycerides that can boost brain function and energy levels, while providing antimicrobial benefits. Both these oils not only add flavor and richness to meals but also offer unique health benefits that support vital bodily functions. By using these nutrient-dense oils in cooking and daily routines, you can effortlessly take a significant step towards a healthier lifestyle.

Olive Oil: Liquid Gold for Longevity

Olive oil, often celebrated as "liquid gold," is a cornerstone of the Mediterranean diet, renowned for its impressive health benefits and potential to boost longevity. Rich in monounsaturated fats and powerful antioxidants like polyphenols, olive oil promotes heart health by reducing inflammation and lowering bad cholesterol levels. Incorporating olive oil into your daily diet isn't just about enhancing flavor; it's about investing in your long-term health. Drizzle it over salads, use it as a base for cooking, or even add a splash to your morning smoothie. These simple acts can help create a shield against chronic diseases, making olive oil an essential addition to a health-focused lifestyle.

Cooking Tips with Olive Oil Olive oil, often referred to as "liquid gold," is a cornerstone of many healthy diets, including the Mediterranean diet, touted for its longevity benefits. But using it effectively requires some knowledge and finesse. While it's famous for its heart-healthy monounsaturated fats and antioxidants, how you cook with olive oil can make a significant difference in both flavor and nutrition.

First and foremost, understanding the types of olive oil available is essential. Extra virgin olive oil (EVOO) is the least processed and retains the most nutrients, whereas virgin olive oil is a slightly refined version with a somewhat milder taste. Then there's regular or pure olive oil, which undergoes more refining and is often mixed with other oils. For everyday cooking, opt for EVOO when you want to preserve as many nutrients and flavors as possible, especially in raw applications like salad dressings or finishing drizzles.

When it comes to cooking methods, using olive oil for sautéing and roasting is an excellent choice. Its smoke point is about 375-410 degrees Fahrenheit (190-210 degrees Celsius), which makes it great for these techniques. However, avoid high-heat methods like deep frying, as olive oil's smoke point is lower than some other oils, and overheating it can produce harmful compounds. Instead, try using EVOO to lightly sauté vegetables or to roast them in the oven. The olive oil not only helps to soften the veggies but also imparts a rich flavor.

One easy way to incorporate olive oil into your daily regimen is by making your own salad dressings. You can whip up a simple vinaigrette using three parts EVOO to one part vinegar, seasoned with salt, pepper, and herbs like basil or oregano. Not only is this healthier than store-bought dressings that often contain preservatives and unhealthy fats, but it also allows you to control the ingredients and flavors. You might even experiment with different vinegars, such as balsamic, red wine, or apple cider vinegar, to keep things interesting.

For those who enjoy baking, olive oil can be a surprising yet delightful substitute for butter or other oils. It works particularly well in Mediterranean-inspired cakes and cookies, imparting a unique depth of flavor along with health benefits. Generally, you can replace butter with olive oil at a 3:4 ratio (use 3/4 cup of olive oil for every 1 cup of butter) in recipes. Try olive oil in a classic olive oil cake with orange zest and almond flour; it's a moist, flavorful alternative that's sure to impress.

Don't overlook olive oil's potential in marinating proteins. It's an excellent base for a marinade mix, helping to tenderize meats while infusing them with flavor. Drizzle olive oil over fish fillets and season with garlic, lemon juice, salt, and pepper for a quick and nutritious meal. Allow it to sit for at least 30 minutes to an hour to let the flavors meld before cooking. This method works particularly well with heart-healthy fish varieties like salmon and mackerel.

Remember, the key to getting the most out of olive oil is not just in its cooking but also its storage. Keep your olive oil in a cool, dark place to protect it from light, air, and heat, all of which can degrade its quality. A tightly sealed container is needed to prevent oxidation. Typically, high-quality olive oil can last up to two years when stored properly, but it's best to use it within a year for optimal flavor and nutrition.

One often overlooked tip is incorporating olive oil into your breakfast routine. A drizzle of EVOO over avocado toast, along with some cherry tomatoes, sprinkled with salt and pepper, makes for a nutrient-dense start to your day. Alternatively, use olive oil to cook your morning eggs. The subtle peppery and fruity notes of the oil can elevate a simple scramble or fried egg to something truly special. This way, you start your day with healthy fats that keep you energized and satiated.

Incorporating olive oil into your diet isn't just about replacing other fats; it's about enhancing the nutrient profile of your meals while amplifying flavors. Take a simple pasta dish to the next level by finishing it with a generous drizzle of EVOO just before serving. This not only adds a layer of complexity to the dish but also aids in the absorption of fat-soluble vitamins present in the vegetables and herbs you're likely pairing with the pasta.

If you're a fan of grilling, brushing vegetables, meats, or fish with olive oil will help prevent sticking while also imparting a delightful flavor. Even fruits like peaches and pineapples benefit from a light coating before they hit the grill. The olive oil helps to caramelize the natural sugars, making for a simple yet sophisticated dessert or salad addition.

Lastly, for a real treat, try infusing your olive oil with different herbs or spices. Infused oils can add an extra dimension to your dishes, whether it's garlic, rosemary, chili, or lemon zest. To make an infused oil, gently heat the olive oil with the desired flavoring until fragrant, then let it cool and strain it into a bottle. Use your infused oils for dressings, marinades, or even a flavorful finishing touch to soups and stews.

Storage: Always store your olive oil in a cool, dark place. This prevents oxidation and maintains its rich flavor.

Smoke Point: Opt for low to medium-heat cooking to preserve the oil's nutrients. High heat can degrade its quality.

Types: Use extra virgin olive oil for salads and finishing, and regular olive oil for cooking.

Baking: Replace butter with olive oil in a 3:4 ratio for healthier baked goods.

Ultimately, whether you're drizzling it over fresh salads, using it as a marinade, or incorporating it into your cooking and baking, olive oil offers countless ways to support your health and longevity. Embrace this versatile, nutrient-dense superfood in your daily culinary practices and experience the myriad benefits it has to offer.

Coconut Oil: A Multipurpose Superfood

Coconut oil has garnered a reputation as a versatile and nutrient-rich addition to the health-conscious pantry. Packed with medium-chain triglycerides (MCTs), it provides a quick source of energy and can assist in weight management by boosting metabolism. Beyond its internal benefits, coconut oil's antifungal and antibacterial properties make it a popular choice for skin and hair care, promoting hydration and healing. Its high smoke point makes it excellent for cooking, ensuring that the nutrients are preserved and harmful compounds are minimized. Whether you're adding it to your morning smoothie, using it as a cooking oil, or applying it topically, coconut oil offers a range of benefits that contribute to overall health and well-being.

Using Coconut Oil in Daily Life is an exciting journey into the versatility and multifaceted applications of this superfood. Coconut oil has earned its rightful place as a staple in kitchens and wellness routines worldwide. Its unique blend of fatty acids, particularly medium-chain triglycerides (MCTs), is what sets it apart as a beneficial addition to your daily life. Whether you're new to coconut oil or already a fan, there's always something new to discover about its myriad uses.

Coconut oil can be a game-changer in the kitchen. Its high smoke point makes it a stellar choice for cooking, sautéing, and even frying, without worrying about harmful oxidation. Imagine whipping up stir-fries, curries, or baking delicious cookies all infused with the subtle, tropical flavor of coconut. For those who love experimenting in the kitchen, coconut oil can replace butter or vegetable oils in most recipes, providing a healthier alternative packed with benefits. Beyond cooking, it also offers an excellent option for greasing baking pans to ensure your baked goods come out perfectly every time.

If you are a smoothie enthusiast, adding a spoonful of coconut oil can give your favorite blends a nutritional boost. Rich in healthy fats, it aids in the absorption of fat-soluble vitamins such as vitamins A, D, E, and K. This makes your nutrient-packed smoothie even more effective. Simply melt the coconut oil slightly, so it integrates seamlessly into cold smoothies without clumping.

Everyday hydration can also be enhanced with coconut oil. Melted and stirred into your morning coffee, it creates a creamy texture and adds to the coffee's richness, acting much like a natural creamer. Known as "Bulletproof Coffee," this combination can provide sustained energy throughout the day and is especially popular among those following ketogenic or low-carb diets.

But the wonders of coconut oil extend far beyond the kitchen. It is a stellar addition to any natural beauty regimen. This oil can serve as a deep-conditioning hair treatment, restoring moisture and shine to lackluster locks. Just warm up a small amount and apply it from the roots to the tips of your hair, leaving it in for at least 30 minutes before washing it out. The result? Soft, manageable, and healthy-looking hair.

For skincare, coconut oil works wonders as a natural moisturizer. It can be applied directly to the skin or mixed with essential oils for added benefits. It's particularly effective for dry or flaky skin, providing a protective barrier that nurtures and heals. If you're into DIY skincare, coconut oil makes an outstanding base for homemade scrubs and salves. Mixing it with sugar or sea salt creates an exfoliating scrub that leaves your skin smooth and refreshed.

Moreover, those who battle with dry or chapped lips can benefit from coconut oil's hydrating properties. Simply dab a little onto your lips for immediate relief, reaping the benefits of its moisturizing qualities without harmful additives found in some commercial lip balms.

In terms of oral care, coconut oil has a long history. One time-honored practice is oil pulling, where you swish a tablespoon of coconut oil in your mouth for about 15-20 minutes. This process can help reduce harmful bacteria and improve overall oral hygiene. It's a simple yet effective routine that can easily be added to your morning regimen.

Coconut oil's antibacterial and antifungal properties make it a natural choice for wound care. Applying a thin layer can help prevent infections and speed up the healing process. It's a gentle option for minor cuts, burns, or insect bites, providing soothing relief and promoting quicker recovery.

If you're a parent, coconut oil can also come in handy for baby care. It's an excellent natural option for diaper rash cream, soothing irritated skin and providing a protective barrier. Applied to dry patches, it can help keep your little one's skin soft and healthy, free from harsh chemicals found in many baby products.

The benefits of coconut oil even extend to our four-legged friends. Pet owners can use coconut oil as a dietary supplement for their pets, promoting a shiny coat and aiding digestion. Applied topically, it can help with skin issues and provide relief from itchy spots, adding an extra layer of care for your furry friends.

When it comes to cleaning, coconut oil shows its versatility yet again. It can be used as a natural wood polish, giving your furniture a beautiful shine. Mixing it with a little lemon juice creates an all-natural cleaner that can make your wooden surfaces glow.

The ingenious uses of coconut oil are nearly limitless, and its benefits positively impacts various facets of daily life. By incorporating coconut oil into both your diet and lifestyle, you are embracing a natural, holistic approach to wellness that nourishes from the inside out. The adaptability of this superfood makes it a worthy addition to anyone's arsenal of health-enhancing tools, perfect for those striving for a balanced, nutrient-rich lifestyle.

Chapter 9:
Berries: The Nutrient-Rich Gems

Berries are nature's potent little packets of nutrition, brimming with antioxidants, vitamins, and fibers that bolster our health remarkably. These tiny gems, whether you favor strawberries, blueberries, raspberries, or blackberries, pack a punch in every bite, helping to improve heart health, boost brain function, and reduce inflammation. Their vibrant colors aren't just a feast for the eyes, but an indication of the treasure trove of anthocyanins and flavonoids contained within. Including berries in your daily diet is a truly delicious way to ensure you get a diverse range of nutrients, making them a cornerstone of any health-conscious regimen. Their versatility in meals—from breakfast bowls and smoothies to salads and desserts—ensures you never grow bored while reaping their myriad health benefits.

Strawberries: Sweet with Benefits

Strawberries are more than just a delicious treat; they are nutritional powerhouses packed with vitamins, antioxidants, and fiber. Among their many benefits, these juicy berries boast high levels of vitamin C, which can boost the immune system, and antioxidants like anthocyanins, which help combat oxidative stress. Consuming strawberries has been linked to improved heart health, reduced inflammation, and even better blood sugar control. Their natural sweetness makes them a versatile addition to any diet, easily incorporated into everything from salads and smoothies to desserts and snacks. Embracing strawberries not only satisfies your sweet tooth but also provides a bounty of health advantages, making them an essential part of a nutrient-rich diet focused on longevity and well-being.

Strawberry-Infused Recipes bring a burst of flavor and nutrition to your meals, making it easier to incorporate this antioxidant-rich fruit into your daily diet. Strawberries are not only deliciously sweet but also pack a significant punch in terms of health benefits. They are full of vitamins, minerals, and antioxidants that support your body in numerous ways. Whether you're looking to boost your immune system, improve heart health, or simply enjoy a tasty treat, strawberries have got you covered.

Let's start with *strawberry salads*. A perfect summer delight, a strawberry spinach salad is both refreshing and nutritious. Combine fresh spinach, sliced strawberries, avocado, walnuts, and feta cheese. Dress this with a simple balsamic vinaigrette made from balsamic vinegar, olive oil, and a touch of honey. This salad is not just a feast for the eyes but also provides a well-rounded mix of vitamins, healthy fats, and proteins.

For those chilly days when you crave something comforting, try *strawberry chia seed pudding*. It's incredibly easy to prepare; mix chia seeds with almond milk and let it sit overnight. In the morning, blend fresh strawberries into a puree and fold it into the pudding. Garnish with a few whole strawberries for extra texture. This pudding is rich in omega-3 fatty acids, protein, and vitamins, a perfect breakfast or snack option to start your day off right.

Another way to enjoy strawberries is *homemade strawberry jam*. Unlike store-bought options that are often laden with sugar, you can control the ingredients and sweetness level. To make, combine fresh strawberries, a bit of honey, and chia seeds in a saucepan. Cook until the strawberries break down and the mixture thickens. Store it in an airtight jar, and it will keep in the fridge for up to two weeks. Spread this low-sugar jam on your morning toast or mix it into yogurt for a wholesome treat.

For a protein-packed option, try a *strawberry smoothie bowl*. Blend strawberries, a banana, Greek yogurt, and a splash of almond milk until smooth. Pour the mixture into a bowl and top with granola, chia seeds, sliced almonds, and more strawberries. This makes for a colorful and nutrient-dense breakfast that's as fun to make as it is delicious to eat.

If you're in the mood for something more indulgent but still healthy, *strawberry chocolate bark* is the way to go. Melt dark chocolate and pour it onto a parchment-lined baking sheet. Sprinkle freeze-dried strawberries and chopped nuts on top. Let it set in the refrigerator until firm, then break into pieces. This treat offers the antioxidant benefits of both dark chocolate and strawberries, making for a guilt-free dessert.

No meal is complete without a refreshing drink, and a *strawberry basil lemonade* is just the ticket. Blend strawberries with fresh lemon juice, a bit of honey, and water. Add a few basil leaves for an unexpected twist that elevates the flavor profile. Serve over ice for a cooling beverage that's perfect on a hot day. This drink is not only hydrating but also brimming with vitamins and antioxidants.

For those special occasions, a *strawberry quinoa salad* makes a great side dish or even a main course. Cook quinoa and let it cool. Add sliced strawberries, cucumber, red onion, feta cheese, and fresh mint. Toss everything in a light lemon dressing for a delightful mix of textures and flavors. This dish is high in protein and fiber, making it a filling and satisfying option.

Desserts are another area where strawberries shine. A *strawberry yogurt parfait* makes for a simple yet delicious dessert. Layer Greek yogurt with strawberry slices and a sprinkle of granola in a glass.

Repeat until you have your desired serving size. Top with a drizzle of honey for added sweetness. This parfait is rich in probiotics, calcium, and antioxidants, offering a healthy way to satisfy your sweet tooth.

Strawberries can also be incorporated into savory dishes. Try making *strawberry salsa* to pair with grilled chicken or fish. Combine diced strawberries, red onion, jalapeno, cilantro, lime juice, and a pinch of salt. The sweetness of the strawberries contrasts beautifully with the heat of the jalapeno and the tanginess of the lime. This salsa is a vibrant, flavorful addition that enhances the nutritional profile of your meal.

Now, let's not forget about breakfast options like *strawberry oatmeal*. Cook your oats as usual, then stir in fresh or frozen strawberries. Top with a handful of nuts and a drizzle of maple syrup for extra flavor. This hearty breakfast is a perfect way to fuel your morning, providing a balanced mix of carbohydrates, protein, and fats.

Another breakfast favorite is *strawberry pancakes*. You can add sliced strawberries directly into the batter or use them as a topping. For a nutrient boost, consider using whole wheat flour or a mix of flours like almond or oat. Serve with a dollop of Greek yogurt and a sprinkling of chia seeds for added texture and nutrition.

Lastly, let's consider *strawberry-infused vinegar*, a wonderful dressing for your salads. Simply combine sliced strawberries and white balsamic vinegar in a jar, seal it, and let it sit for a week in the refrigerator. Strain out the strawberries before using. This infused vinegar not only enhances the taste of your salads but also offers additional health benefits.

Overall, **strawberry-infused recipes** can transform ordinary meals into extraordinary ones. Their versatility and nutritional prowess make strawberries a worthy addition to your superfood repertoire. From breakfast to dessert and everything in between, these recipes demonstrate that eating healthy can be both delicious and easy. Embrace the sweet, vibrant nature of strawberries and let them add a burst of flavor and nourishment to your daily meals.

Raspberries: Antioxidant Rich

Raspberries, those vibrant red gems, are a powerhouse of antioxidants, notably ellagic acid, quercetin, and vitamin C. These compounds are essential for neutralizing free radicals, which can help reduce oxidative stress and inflammation in the body. Regular consumption of raspberries may improve heart health, support cognitive function, and even contribute to cancer prevention. Their high fiber content also promotes healthy digestion and helps regulate blood sugar levels. With a delightful combination of sweetness and tartness, raspberries are not only a nutritional asset but also a versatile ingredient that can elevate both savory and sweet dishes, making it easy to integrate these nutrient-dense berries into your everyday diet.

Boosting Meals with Raspberries brings an array of fresh flavors and nutrition to your diet. Often overlooked due to their delicate texture and seasonal availability, raspberries are a treasure trove of health benefits. This tiny superfood packs a big punch when it comes to nutrients and can be effortlessly integrated into a variety of meals. But what makes raspberries so special, and how can you take advantage of their superfood status?

First, let's delve into the nutrient profile of raspberries. These berries are rich in fiber, antioxidants, vitamins, and minerals. One cup of raspberries contains about 8 grams of dietary fiber, making up around 32% of the daily recommended intake for adults. Fiber is essential for digestion and can help in regulating blood sugar levels and reducing cholesterol.

Beyond their fiber content, raspberries also provide a high dose of vitamin C and manganese, along with smaller amounts of vitamin K, vitamin E, folate, and iron. These nutrients collectively contribute to immune function, skin health, and bone strength. With such a rich nutrient profile, raspberries are indeed a powerhouse of health benefits.

Antioxidants are another significant component of raspberries. These compounds help combat oxidative stress and inflammation in the body, providing protection against chronic diseases such as heart disease, diabetes, and even cancer. The key antioxidants in raspberries include quercetin, ellagic acid, and anthocyanins, responsible for their deep red color. Incorporating raspberries into your meals can significantly boost your antioxidant intake, offering you a natural defense mechanism.

Now, let's explore how to effortlessly integrate raspberries into your daily meals. Breakfast is a fantastic time to start, and a raspberry-infused smoothie can be both nutritious and delicious. Combine a handful of raspberries with some Greek yogurt, a banana, a spoonful of almond butter, and a splash of almond milk for a creamy, nutrient-packed start to your day. You can also add chia seeds or flaxseeds for an extra fiber and omega-3 boost.

If smoothies aren't your thing, don't worry! Raspberries are incredibly versatile and can be added to oatmeal, yogurt bowls, or even mixed into pancake or waffle batter. For a quick and healthy breakfast option, try stirring raspberries into your overnight oats along with some chopped nuts and a drizzle of honey. The natural sweetness of the berries will blend perfectly with the rich, creamy texture of the oats.

Moving on to lunch, raspberry vinaigrette is a game-changer. This tangy, sweet dressing can transform any salad into a gourmet meal. Blend fresh raspberries with olive oil, apple cider vinegar, a touch of honey, and a pinch of salt and pepper. Drizzle it over a mixed greens salad with goat cheese, walnuts, and grilled chicken for a dish bursting with flavors and nutrients.

Raspberries can also be a fantastic addition to grain bowls. Combine cooked quinoa with diced cucumbers, cherry tomatoes, avocado, spinach, and a handful of raspberries for a refreshing, filling meal. The berries add a delightful pop of color and sweetness, making every bite a treat.

Dinner offers even more opportunities to include these nutrient-rich gems. Consider making a raspberry glaze for your protein. Whether it's chicken, pork, or tofu, a raspberry glaze can add a luxurious touch. To make it, simmer fresh raspberries with balsamic vinegar, a bit of honey, and some fresh rosemary. Let it reduce to a syrupy consistency, then brush it over your protein of choice. The result is a dish that's both elegant and healthy, with the raspberries' natural sweetness perfectly complementing the savory notes of the protein.

For those who enjoy baking, raspberries can elevate your homemade bread or muffins. Mixing them into the batter can add bursts of flavor and nutrition. Try making raspberry-almond muffins with whole wheat flour, using honey or maple syrup as a natural sweetener. The combination of raspberries and almonds not only tastes incredible but also offers a significant nutritional benefit, including antioxidants and healthy fats.

Raspberries make an excellent addition to desserts, too. A raspberry chia pudding can be an incredibly healthy yet indulgent treat. Blend raspberries with almond milk, add chia seeds, and allow the mixture to set in the fridge for a few hours. Before serving, top it with more fresh raspberries and a sprinkle of shredded coconut. This dessert is not only delicious but also high in fiber, omega-3s, and antioxidants.

If you're feeling adventurous, you can even use raspberries in savory dishes. Try adding them to a socca (a chickpea flour flatbread) with some caramelized onions and a sprinkle of goat cheese. Another option is a raspberry salsa, made by combining diced mango, red onion, jalapeño, cilantro, and raspberries. This can be served with grilled fish or as a topping for tacos, adding a unique twist to your meal.

Don't forget the beverages! Raspberry-infused drinks are both refreshing and good for you. Make a raspberry mint cooler by muddling fresh raspberries with mint leaves, adding sparkling water, and a squeeze of lime. It's a perfect way to stay hydrated while enjoying a burst of flavor and getting some extra nutrients.

Incorporating raspberries into your meals doesn't have to be complicated. A simple handful sprinkled over your cereal, mixed into your salads, or added to a dessert recipe can make a significant difference to your health. It's all about finding small, manageable ways to integrate these superfoods into your existing diet.

Remember, the key to maximizing the health benefits of raspberries is consistency. They offer a plethora of nutrients and antioxidants that can't be fully harnessed unless consumed regularly. By making raspberries a staple in your kitchen, you ensure that you're always just a step away from a nutrient-rich, antioxidant-packed meal.

So, go ahead and start experimenting. The versatility of raspberries means you'll never run out of ways to enjoy them. From breakfasts to dinners, snacks to desserts, there's always a place for these vibrant, health-boosting gems in your diet.

Chapter 10:
Vegetables

Incorporating a variety of vegetables into your daily diet is one of the most powerful ways to enhance your health and longevity. Vegetables like sweet potatoes and broccoli aren't just side dishes; they're nutritional powerhouses packed with essential vitamins, minerals, and fiber. Sweet potatoes, with their rich beta-carotene content, support eye health and immune function, while broccoli's cruciferous compounds have been shown to reduce inflammation and improve detoxification. The vibrant colors of these vegetables aren't just pleasing to the eye; they signify an abundance of phytonutrients that work synergistically to protect your cells and promote overall wellbeing. By making vegetables a mainstay of your meals, you create a foundation for a diet that's as healing as it is delicious, paving the way for longer, healthier life.

Sweet Potatoes: Nutritional Powerhouses

Sweet potatoes, with their vibrant orange hue, are more than just a versatile culinary ingredient; they are a rich source of essential nutrients that can significantly boost your health. Packed with beta-carotene, which the body converts to vitamin A, sweet potatoes support vision, immune function, and skin health. Additionally, they're high in dietary fiber, which aids digestion and helps maintain stable blood sugar levels. These tubers are also loaded with vitamins C and E, crucial for their antioxidant properties, reducing inflammation, and promoting healthy aging. Incorporating sweet potatoes into your diet doesn't require complex recipes—roasting, baking, or mashing them can turn this nutritional powerhouse into a delicious and health-boosting meal component.

Sweet Potato Recipes for All Meals are a delightful way to make the most of this versatile, nutrient-packed vegetable. Sweet potatoes are high in fiber, vitamins, and minerals, making them an excellent choice for those looking to boost their health and longevity. With their natural sweetness and satisfying texture, they can be incorporated into every meal of the day, offering endless possibilities for delicious and nutritious dishes. Let's dive into some creative recipes that demonstrate the incredible range of sweet potatoes.

Starting with breakfast, sweet potatoes can form the base of a satisfying morning meal. Consider sweet potato pancakes, a healthy twist on the traditional breakfast favorite. To prepare, grate peeled sweet potatoes and mix with flour, eggs, and a dash of cinnamon. Heat a skillet and cook until golden brown, then top with fresh berries and a drizzle of honey.

If you prefer savory mornings, sweet potato hash is another great option. Dice sweet potatoes into small cubes and sauté them with onions, bell peppers, and your favorite seasoning. Top with fried eggs for a protein-rich breakfast that's both filling and flavorful.

For a quick weekday lunch, sweet potato and black bean burritos can be your go-to. Simply roast diced sweet potatoes with cumin and chili powder, then combine with black beans, avocado, and salsa. Wrap everything in a whole-grain tortilla for a nutrient-dense meal that's easy to take on the go. The creamy texture of the avocado paired with the slightly spicy roasted sweet potatoes creates a satisfying combination that'll keep you energized throughout the afternoon.

Sweet potatoes also shine in soups and stews. Their natural sweetness and robustness make them ideal for hearty lunchtime dishes. A sweet potato and lentil soup is warming and rich, perfect for those cooler days. Start by sautéing onions and garlic, then add diced sweet potatoes, lentils, and vegetable broth. Let it simmer until everything is tender. Season it with turmeric and cumin for a warming, anti-inflammatory kick.

Dinner is where sweet potatoes can truly be the star. Think about a nourishing sweet potato and chickpea curry. Cut sweet potatoes into chunks and cook them with chickpeas, coconut milk, tomatoes, and a mix of spices like curry powder and garam masala. Serve over quinoa or brown rice to soak up every bit of the delicious sauce. This dish not only tastes wonderful but is also incredibly nutrient-dense, aligning perfectly with a health-focused lifestyle.

For a more traditional take on sweet potatoes at dinner, try them roasted with a variety of herbs. Simply toss sweet potato wedges in olive oil, salt, pepper, and rosemary. Roast at a high temperature until crispy on the outside and tender on the inside. These can be a perfect side to roasted chicken or a hearty salad.

Sweet potatoes can even make their way into your dessert menu. Sweet potato pie is a classic, but consider a healthier twist with sweet potato brownies. Blend mashed sweet potatoes with cacao powder, almond flour, and a natural sweetener like maple syrup. Bake until firm and enjoy these guilt-free treats that are rich in antioxidants and fiber.

Another creative dessert idea is sweet potato pudding. Combine cooked, mashed sweet potatoes with coconut milk, cinnamon, nutmeg, and a splash of vanilla extract. Chill in the refrigerator and serve topped with crushed nuts or a sprinkle of coconut flakes. This creamy, luscious pudding can satisfy your sweet tooth while providing a nutrient boost.

Don't forget about sweet potato snacks. Sweet potato chips are a fantastic, healthy alternative to store-bought versions. Thinly slice sweet potatoes and lightly coat with olive oil and sea salt. Bake until crispy for a delightful snack that's both crunchy and nutritious. Especially when paired with a homemade guacamole or a roasted red pepper dip, these chips can become a staple in your snack rotation.

You can even integrate sweet potatoes into salads for added flavor and nutrient variety. A roasted sweet potato and kale salad packs a punch of vitamins and minerals. Toss chopped sweet potatoes with olive oil and your favorite seasoning, then roast until tender. Add to a bowl of massaged kale, quinoa, dried cranberries, and pecans. Dress with a lemon-tahini dressing for a truly vibrant dish that works well as a main course or side.

For those who enjoy meal prepping, sweet potatoes are incredibly versatile and can be made in advance. Prepare a large batch of roasted sweet potatoes at the beginning of the week, and you'll find countless ways to incorporate them into your meals. Whether adding them to a grain bowl, mixing into an omelet, or combining with beans for a quick quesadilla filling, roasted sweet potatoes can enhance many dishes.

The possibilities are, indeed, endless when it comes to sweet potatoes. They adapt well to various cooking methods and flavors, ensuring you can continually experiment and enjoy them in new ways. Utilizing sweet potatoes across breakfast, lunch, dinner, snacks, and even desserts maximizes their potential as a superfood in your diet.

By incorporating these recipes into your regular meal rotation, you can not only enjoy the delicious taste of sweet potatoes but also harness their substantial health benefits. Loaded with vitamins like A and C, fiber, potassium, and antioxidants, sweet potatoes contribute significantly to your overall well-being and longevity. Experimenting with sweet potatoes in different meals underlines the versatility and unmatched potential of this humble vegetable.

Broccoli: The Cruciferous Champion

Broccoli, often hailed as a nutritional powerhouse, stands out as a quintessential superfood in the vegetable kingdom. Rich in vitamins such as C and K, and brimming with fiber, this green gem offers an array of health benefits that can significantly boost your well-being. Its antioxidant properties combat oxidative stress, reducing inflammation and supporting heart health. Sulforaphane, a compound found in broccoli, has been studied for its role in cancer prevention. Additionally, this versatile cruciferous vegetable can be easily incorporated into a variety of dishes, from stir-fries and salads to soups and casseroles, making it an accessible and delicious way to enhance your diet. By integrating broccoli into your meals, you're not just adding flavor, but also investing in a longer, healthier life.

Broccoli in Everyday Cooking is about more than just a side dish; it's about integrating a nutrient-dense superfood into your daily culinary repertoire. With its high levels of vitamins C, K, and A, as well as fiber and a range of antioxidants, broccoli offers numerous health benefits that can support your overall wellness and longevity. But how do you make this green vegetable a staple in your meals without it becoming monotonous?

First off, let's get to the basics—steaming. For many, this is the simplest method to prepare broccoli. Steamed broccoli is incredibly versatile and can be an excellent addition to salads, pastas, or even as a standalone side dish. Just add a squeeze of lemon, a drizzle of olive oil, and a sprinkle of sea salt to enhance its natural flavors. Steaming preserves most of the vegetables' nutrients, ensuring you receive its full health benefits.

Roasting, on the other hand, brings out broccoli's sweeter, nuttier side. To roast broccoli, toss the florets with some olive oil, minced garlic, and a bit of salt and pepper. Then, spread them out on a baking sheet and cook at 425°F (220°C) until they are tender and slightly crispy at the edges, usually around 20-25 minutes. The high heat caramelizes the edges, adding a delicious depth to their flavor.

Broccoli rice has gained popularity as a low-carb, nutrient-packed alternative to traditional rice. To make broccoli rice, simply pulse the florets in a food processor until they reach a rice-like consistency. Sauté the "rice" in a pan with some olive oil, garlic, and a bit of salt. This can be particularly useful for those looking to reduce their carbohydrate intake without compromising on nutrition.

Incorporating broccoli into soups is another fantastic way to enjoy its benefits. A creamy broccoli soup made with cashews or coconut milk can provide a rich, satisfying meal that's both dairy-free and bursting with flavor. Simply sauté onions and garlic, add chopped broccoli and broth, then simmer until the broccoli is tender. Blend the mixture until smooth, and stir in your choice of cream substitute for a velvety texture.

Let's not forget about stir-fries. Broccoli's firm texture holds up well in high-heat cooking, making it perfect for a quick and nutritious stir-fry. Combine broccoli with other vegetables like bell peppers, snap peas, and carrots. Add tofu, chicken, or shrimp for protein, and toss everything in a savory sauce made from soy sauce, ginger, and garlic. Serve over whole grains like quinoa or brown rice for a complete meal.

Sometimes, simplicity is key. A straightforward broccoli salad can make for an easy, make-ahead lunch or dinner side. Combine blanched broccoli florets with red onions, sunflower seeds, and dried cranberries. For the dressing, mix Greek yogurt with apple cider vinegar, honey, and a touch of mustard. This recipe is as quick as it is delicious, and it can be stored in the fridge for days without losing its crisp texture.

Broccoli can also shine in more unconventional recipes. Think of broccoli in a smoothie! It might sound odd at first, but when blended with fruits like pineapple and mango, the broccoli becomes nearly undetectable, creating a nutrient-rich, green smoothie that's perfect for a morning boost.

For those who love pasta, don't overlook the potential of broccoli in pasta dishes. A garlic, broccoli, and lemon pasta can be a zesty, nutrient-packed meal. Start by steaming or boiling the broccoli until just tender. Meanwhile, cook your favorite pasta. In another pan, sauté garlic in olive oil, then add the cooked broccoli and cooked pasta. Squeeze fresh lemon juice over the top and toss everything together with a sprinkling of Parmesan cheese.

Pizza and broccoli? Absolutely. Add steamed or roasted broccoli to your pizza toppings for an extra dose of greens. Broccoli pairs beautifully with flavors like roasted red peppers, olives, and feta cheese. Whether you're making a homemade dough or using a whole-grain store-bought crust, adding broccoli can boost the nutrition content of your pizza night exponentially.

Even breakfast can be a time to include broccoli. Consider a vegetable-packed frittata or omelet. Simply sauté some chopped broccoli along with onions, peppers, and any other favorite veggies, then pour beaten eggs over the mixture. Cook on the stovetop until the edges are set, then finish it off in the oven. It's an easy, make-ahead breakfast that's both satisfying and nutrient-packed.

Broccoli slaw is a great way to use the often-overlooked broccoli stems. Shred the stems and combine them with shredded carrots and cabbage. Toss with a dressing made from Greek yogurt, apple cider vinegar, and a bit of honey. This crisp, tangy slaw is perfect for sandwiches, as a taco topping, or simply as a refreshing side dish.

Integrating broccoli into casseroles can transform these comforting, often calorie-dense dishes into healthier options. Mix steamed broccoli into classics like macaroni and cheese or a rice and chicken casserole. The added fiber and vitamins from the broccoli enhance the dish's nutritional profile without compromising its comforting nature.

During summer months, consider grilling broccoli. Grilled broccoli offers a smoky flavor that pairs wonderfully with summer barbecues. Simply coat the florets in olive oil, season with salt and pepper, and grill until tender and charred in spots. Serve with a squeeze of lemon juice and a sprinkle of Parmesan for an easy side dish.

Don't underestimate broccoli as a potent ingredient in dips. A broccoli and cheddar dip can be both healthy and satisfying. Steam broccoli until tender, then blend it with cheddar cheese, Greek yogurt, and a touch of garlic powder. Serve with whole-grain crackers or vegetable sticks for a nutrient-rich snack.

Finally, consider the global culinary stage for inspiration. In Asian cuisine, broccoli is a staple in many dishes. In Indian cuisine, you might find it in curries with spices like turmeric and cumin. In Italian cooking, broccoli rabe, which is closely related to broccoli, is often paired with garlic and olive oil in simple yet delicious preparations. Exploring these global approaches can add variety and excitement to your daily meals.

By creatively incorporating broccoli into various dishes throughout the day, you can ensure you're taking full advantage of its incredible health benefits. Whether it's through simple preparations or creative culinary twists, making broccoli a regular part of your daily diet can contribute significantly to your health and longevity goals. Bon appétit!

Chapter 11:
Superfood Spices

The potent power of spices extends well beyond flavor enhancement—they're small but mighty contributors to health and longevity. Take turmeric, for instance. Known as the "golden spice," it boasts curcumin, a compound with powerful anti-inflammatory and antioxidant properties. Ginger, another profound player, not only adds a fragrant zest but also aids digestion, reduces nausea, and helps fight chronic inflammation. By incorporating these superfood spices into your daily diet, you can transform everyday meals into culinary experiences while boosting your health in numerous ways. These spices are easy to integrate into a wide variety of dishes, making them both accessible and versatile tools for enhancing wellness.

Turmeric: The Golden Spice

Turmeric, often hailed as the "Golden Spice," is a powerhouse of health benefits that can significantly enhance your well-being when incorporated into your daily regimen. Known for its vibrant yellow hue and distinct flavor, turmeric's active compound, curcumin, boasts potent anti-inflammatory and antioxidant properties. These attributes not only assist in combating chronic inflammation but may also lower the risk of various diseases, including heart disease and cancer. Adding turmeric to your diet is straightforward and versatile; it can be mixed into smoothies, sprinkled over roasted vegetables, or even brewed into a soothing tea. By embracing the golden spice, you're not just adding a burst of flavor to your meals—you're investing in your health and longevity.

Turmeric-Infused Recipes is one of the most vibrant superfood spices, commonly recognized by its bright yellow hue and earthy aroma. This golden spice, derived from the root of the Curcuma longa plant, is not just a staple in Indian cuisine but is also celebrated globally for its potential health benefits. The primary active compound in turmeric, curcumin, is known for its powerful anti-inflammatory and antioxidant properties, making turmeric a nutrient-dense addition to anyone's diet.

Integrating turmeric into your daily meals doesn't have to be a challenge. One simple and delicious way to start is with *Golden Milk*. This warm, soothing beverage combines turmeric with milk (dairy or plant-based), a sprinkle of black pepper, and optional spices like cinnamon and ginger. The black pepper is crucial as it enhances the absorption of curcumin, amplifying turmeric's health benefits. To prepare Golden Milk, gently heat 2 cups of milk with 1 teaspoon of turmeric, 1/2 teaspoon of cinnamon, a pinch of black pepper, and add a sweetener like honey to taste. Simmer for a few minutes, strain, and enjoy this comforting drink as a morning boost or nighttime relaxant.

For a savory option, consider making *Turmeric and Ginger Roasted Vegetables*. This dish showcases the versatility of turmeric in everyday cooking. Toss your favorite vegetables—carrots, sweet potatoes, and cauliflower work wonderfully—with olive oil, turmeric, freshly grated ginger, garlic, salt, and pepper. Roast at 400°F for about 25-30 minutes until tender and caramelized. The result is a visually appealing, nutrient-packed side dish that pairs well with any main course.

If you're a fan of curries, you'll love *Turmeric Chickpea Curry*. This vegetarian dish combines protein-rich chickpeas with the flavor and health benefits of turmeric. Sauté chopped onions, garlic, and ginger in coconut oil until fragrant. Add in 1 tablespoon of turmeric, 2 teaspoons of cumin, 1 teaspoon of coriander, and a pinch of cayenne pepper. Stir in a can of coconut milk and a can of diced tomatoes, then add two cans of drained and rinsed chickpeas. Simmer for about 20 minutes, allowing the flavors to meld together. Serve this curry over a bed of quinoa or brown rice for a complete, nutrient-dense meal.

For those who enjoy baking, *Turmeric Banana Bread* is an excellent way to sneak this superfood into your diet. This recipe adds a unique twist to traditional banana bread, infusing it with the subtle warmth of turmeric. In a large bowl, mash three ripe bananas and mix with 1/3 cup melted coconut oil, 1 teaspoon of vanilla extract, and 1/2 cup of honey or maple syrup. In a separate bowl, blend 1 1/2 cups of whole wheat flour, 1 teaspoon of baking soda, 1 teaspoon of turmeric, and a pinch of salt. Combine the wet and dry ingredients, pour into a greased loaf pan, and bake at 350°F for 50-60 minutes. This turmeric banana bread makes for a nourishing breakfast or snack.

Another delightful treat is *Turmeric and Lemon Energy Balls*. These no-bake snacks are perfect for a quick boost of energy and nutrition. In a food processor, combine 1 cup of pitted dates, 1 cup of almonds, 2 tablespoons of coconut oil, 1 teaspoon of turmeric, 1 teaspoon of fresh lemon zest, and a pinch of salt. Blend until the mixture sticks together. Roll into bite-sized balls and refrigerate for at least an hour to firm up. These energy balls are not only convenient for a quick snack but also a tasty way to incorporate turmeric into your day.

Soups can also benefit from the addition of turmeric. A *Turmeric Lentil Soup* is both hearty and healing. Start by sautéing diced onions, carrots, and celery in olive oil until softened. Add minced garlic, 1 teaspoon of turmeric, 1 teaspoon of cumin, and 1 teaspoon of coriander, cooking for another minute. Stir in 1 cup of red lentils, 4 cups of vegetable broth, and a can of diced tomatoes. Bring to a boil, then reduce the heat and simmer for 20-25 minutes until the lentils are tender. Finish with a squeeze of lemon juice and a handful of fresh spinach for added nutrients.

For a refreshing salad, try a *Turmeric Quinoa Salad*. Cook 1 cup of quinoa according to package instructions, adding 1 teaspoon of turmeric to the cooking water. Once cooked and cooled, toss the quinoa with chopped cucumber, cherry tomatoes, red onion, and fresh herbs like parsley or cilantro. Dress the salad with a mixture of olive oil, lemon juice, salt, and pepper. This vibrant salad is not only visually appealing but also packed with health-promoting properties.

Breakfast options can also be enhanced with turmeric. One such recipe is *Turmeric-Spiced Overnight Oats*. In a jar, combine 1/2 cup of rolled oats, 1/2 cup of almond milk, 1/2 teaspoon of turmeric, 1/4 teaspoon of cinnamon, a pinch of black pepper, and a tablespoon of chia seeds. Stir well, cover, and refrigerate overnight. In the morning, top with fresh berries, a drizzle of honey, and a sprinkle of nuts for a nourishing and easy start to your day.

Golden Milk - A warm, soothing beverage with turmeric and spices.

Turmeric and Ginger Roasted Vegetables - A savory side dish with roasted vegetables.

Turmeric Chickpea Curry - A vegetarian curry with chickpeas and coconut milk.

Turmeric Banana Bread - A unique twist on traditional banana bread with added turmeric.

Turmeric and Lemon Energy Balls - No-bake snacks infused with turmeric and lemon zest.

Turmeric Lentil Soup - A hearty and healing soup with lentils and vegetables.

Turmeric Quinoa Salad - A vibrant salad with quinoa, vegetables, and herbs.

Turmeric-Spiced Overnight Oats - A convenient breakfast option with oats and turmeric.

Turmeric Hummus is another great way to add this superfood to your diet. Blend a can of chickpeas, 1/4 cup of tahini, 2 tablespoons of olive oil, the juice of one lemon, 1-2 cloves of garlic, 1 teaspoon of turmeric, and a pinch of salt in a food processor until smooth. This vibrant hummus is perfect as a dip or spread, adding a

Ginger: Spice and Everything Nice

Ginger is more than just a zesty addition to your favorite dishes; it's a nutritional powerhouse with a rich history in both culinary and medicinal traditions. This spicy root is packed with bioactive compounds, notably gingerol, which has potent anti-inflammatory and antioxidant effects. Regular consumption of ginger can aid digestion, reduce nausea, and combat chronic conditions like hypertension and heart disease. Whether you're grating it fresh into a smoothie, adding it to your stir-fries, or sipping on ginger tea, incorporating ginger into your daily routine can significantly boost your overall health and longevity. It's a simple yet effective way to harness the power of superfood spices for a healthier life.

Creative Uses for Ginger Ginger is not just a spice to add a zesty kick to your meals – it's a versatile superfood that can truly revolutionize your culinary experience while boosting your health. Known for its distinct flavor and potent anti-inflammatory properties, ginger offers a plethora of uses that extend beyond traditional kitchen borders. From revitalizing beverages to savory dishes, let's explore innovative ways to incorporate ginger into your everyday routine.

One of the simplest yet highly effective ways to enjoy ginger's benefits is by making ginger tea. Just slice a piece of fresh ginger, about the size of your thumb, and steep it in hot water for 5-10 minutes. Both soothing and invigorating, ginger tea can help combat nausea, improve digestion, and even reduce muscle pain after a workout. You can also enhance the flavor and health benefits by adding a dash of lemon juice and honey. This drink proves that sometimes the most beneficial remedies are also the simplest.

Another creative use for ginger is in smoothies. A small piece of fresh or a pinch of ground ginger can add a refreshing zing to fruit and vegetable blends. For instance, combine ginger with pineapple, spinach, and coconut water for a tropical smoothie that's not only delicious but also packed with vitamins and antioxidants. This blend is perfect for kickstarting your day with an energy boost or as a rejuvenating post-workout drink.

Ginger's flavor profile makes it an excellent addition to both savory and sweet dishes. For savory applications, consider creating a ginger-infused marinade for proteins like chicken, tofu, or fish. A marinade made from soy sauce, minced garlic, fresh ginger, and a bit of sesame oil will impart a rich, savory taste that's hard to resist. Let your chosen protein soak in this flavorful concoction for at least 30 minutes before cooking to ensure the ginger's essence is deeply absorbed.

In the realm of sweets, ginger pairs exceptionally well with desserts. Gingerbread cookies and ginger snaps are classic examples, but don't stop there. Try adding grated ginger to your apple pie filling for a warm, spicy twist that enhances the fruit's natural sweetness. Alternatively, ginger can be used in making homemade granola or energy bars. Simply mix oats, nuts, honey, and finely chopped ginger before baking. The result will be a snack that's both satisfying and nutritious.

For those looking to add a gourmet touch to their meals, ginger can be pickled, candied, or even used to create a ginger syrup. Pickled ginger, often seen accompanying sushi, is excellent for adding a tart, spicy element to salads and sandwiches. Candied ginger, on the other hand, serves as a delightful topping for yogurt, oatmeal, or ice cream. Creating ginger syrup is straightforward and yields a versatile ingredient you can use to sweeten drinks, flavor pancakes, or drizzle over fruit salads. To make ginger syrup, simmer equal parts water and sugar with sliced ginger until the liquid thickens to your desired consistency. Strain out the ginger pieces and let the syrup cool before storing it in the fridge.

In culinary traditions worldwide, ginger takes on a unique role in enhancing flavors. For example, in Indian cuisine, ginger-garlic paste is a staple ingredient used in numerous dishes. Combining equal parts of ginger and garlic in a food processor creates a paste that can be frozen in small portions and added to curries, stews, and stir-fries. This paste not only adds a robust flavor but also brings the digestive and immune-boosting benefits of both ginger and garlic to your meals.

Ginger's pungent and somewhat sweet taste also makes it an ideal ingredient for creating unique beverages. Beyond the classic ginger tea, try crafting your own ginger beer or ginger-infused lemonade. Homemade ginger beer involves fermenting ginger, sugar, water, and a culture called a ginger bug, resulting in a fizzy, probiotic-rich drink. Ginger lemonade, made by mixing lemon juice, ginger syrup, and water, is a refreshing beverage that's perfect for summer or whenever you need a revitalizing lift.

In the world of soups and broths, ginger's warmth and spice come into their own. Adding fresh slices of ginger to chicken or vegetable broths can elevate the flavor while adding anti-inflammatory and immune-supporting properties. A ginger-carrot soup, blending the sweetness of carrots with the spice of ginger, makes for a comforting and nutrient-rich dish. Similarly, coconut-ginger soup, a creamy and aromatic recipe common in Thai cuisine, balances spices and creaminess beautifully.

Don't overlook the potential of ginger in baked goods. Besides the familiar gingerbread and ginger snaps, ginger can also enhance banana bread, muffins, and cakes. Just a teaspoon of ground ginger or a tablespoon of freshly grated ginger can transform an ordinary batter into something extraordinary, providing an unexpected twist that delights the palate.

For those engaged in fitness and needing a recovery boost, ginger can be incorporated into quick, protein-rich snacks. Combining mashed chickpeas, oats, ginger, and other spices can create energy balls that are perfect for a pre-workout snack or a post-exercise recovery treat. These snacks offer a balance of protein, carbs, and anti-inflammatory compounds, helping your body recover faster.

Intertwined with ginger's diverse culinary applications are its numerous health benefits. Regularly incorporating ginger into your diet can improve digestion, reduce nausea, fight inflammation, and even lower blood sugar levels. The root's high levels of gingerol, a compound with powerful medicinal properties, underscore ginger's status as a superfood.

Lastly, consider the aesthetic and sensory experience that ginger can bring to your dishes. Its distinctive aroma, visual appeal, and complex flavor profile can elevate the simplest meal into a gourmet experience. Sprinkle finely chopped fresh ginger over roasted vegetables or mix ground ginger into spice rubs for meat and fish. The possibilities are virtually endless, and experimentation can lead to delightful culinary discoveries.

Incorporating ginger into your daily life doesn't have to be complex. Start small, perhaps by adding a pinch of ginger powder to your morning oatmeal or blending a slice of fresh ginger into your smoothie. As you grow more comfortable with this versatile root, you'll find countless ways to enjoy its flavors and health benefits.

So, whether you're a seasoned chef or a kitchen novice, ginger provides an easy and delicious gateway to healthier eating. With its robust flavor and remarkable versatility, this modest root can truly transform your meals and, notably, your overall well-being.

Chapter 12:
Adaptogens

Adaptogens, often heralded as nature's miracle workers, are unique botanical compounds that help the body resist and recover from physical, mental, and emotional stress. These powerful herbs and roots, including ashwagandha, maca, and rhodiola, have been utilized for centuries across various cultures for their remarkable ability to restore balance and enhance resilience. Adaptogens support homeostasis by modulating hormone production, improving energy levels, and boosting the immune system. Through their multifaceted benefits, they offer an invaluable resource for anyone aiming to achieve optimal health amidst the demands of modern life. Incorporating adaptogens into your daily routine could be the key to unlocking newfound vitality and longevity.

Ashwagandha: The Stress Reliever

Ashwagandha, often hailed as one of the most powerful adaptogens, has been celebrated for its remarkable ability to help our bodies manage stress. This ancient herb, rooted in Ayurvedic medicine, doesn't just soothe the mind; it also promotes overall well-being by balancing cortisol levels, enhancing mental clarity, and boosting energy. Incorporating ashwagandha into your daily routine is simple and can be as easy as adding its powdered form to your morning smoothie or evening tea. Its adaptogenic properties help modulate the body's response to stress while supporting immune function, making it an invaluable addition to any health-focused lifestyle.

Adding Ashwagandha to Your Daily Routine is a highly beneficial practice, given its wide range of health properties. This adaptogen, commonly referred to as Indian ginseng or winter cherry, has taken the wellness community by storm, and for good reason. Integrating ashwagandha into your daily routine can help in managing stress, enhancing cognitive function, and boosting overall vitality. To harness these benefits fully, the first step is understanding how to seamlessly incorporate this versatile herb into various aspects of your life.

This powerful root can be used in multiple ways, thanks to its adaptability in both dietary and supplemental forms. One of the simplest methods to include ashwagandha is by using powder form, which can be added to smoothies, teas, and even coffee. Many prefer taking it in capsule form for convenience, ensuring they receive a consistent dosage without altering their meals.

Incorporating ashwagandha into your meals can be a delightful experience. If you're a smoothie enthusiast, adding a teaspoon of ashwagandha powder to your blend of fruits, greens, and plant-based milk can provide an additional wellness boost without compromising flavor. Some people even mix it into their morning oatmeal or soups. Just a small amount can impact your energy levels and stress resilience throughout the day.

For those who enjoy teas, ashwagandha can be brewed as an herbal tea. Simply mix the powder with hot water and let it steep for a few minutes. You might consider adding a bit of honey or lemon to enhance the taste, making it a comforting and health-enhancing ritual in your daily routine. If you enjoy experimenting, creating an ashwagandha latte with almond milk, a dash of cinnamon, and a touch of vanilla can turn this adaptogen into a gourmet experience.

Beyond culinary uses, another convenient option for incorporating ashwagandha into your routine is through supplements. Available in various forms such as capsules, tinctures, and even gummies, supplements can provide a consistent and measured dose of this potent herb. Always ensure you're purchasing from a reputable brand to guarantee quality and purity. It's advisable to follow the recommended dosage listed on the product or consult with a healthcare professional to tailor it to your specific needs.

Ashwagandha's flexibility doesn't end there. Combining it with other superfoods can amplify its benefits. Pairing ashwagandha with turmeric in a golden milk recipe, for instance, not only boosts the anti-inflammatory properties of both herbs but also creates a soothing nighttime beverage. This combination can be particularly beneficial for those looking to enhance sleep quality and reduce evening stress.

When adding ashwagandha to your daily routine, consistency is key. Like many natural supplements, the effects of ashwagandha build up over time, so it's essential to make it a regular part of your lifestyle. Many users report noticing significant improvements in their stress levels, energy, and overall wellness after consistently including ashwagandha in their regimen for several weeks.

Finding the optimal time of day to take ashwagandha can vary depending on your personal needs and lifestyle. Some prefer taking it in the morning to start the day with a calm and focused mind, while others favor an evening dose to unwind and promote restful sleep. Experiment with timing to discover what works best for you.

However, it's not just about timing; dosage plays a crucial role as well. The typical dosage ranges from 300 to 500 mg of standardized root extract per day, but this can differ based on individual health conditions and goals. Lower dosages might be effective for mild stress relief, whereas higher dosages may be necessary for chronic conditions or more substantial health goals. Consulting with a healthcare provider can tailor the right dosage to maximize benefits while avoiding potential adverse effects.

In addition to its stress-relieving properties, ashwagandha has a positive impact on physical performance and muscle strength. For those who lead an active lifestyle or engage in regular exercise, incorporating ashwagandha can lead to improved stamina and potentially better workout results. Including it in a pre- or post-workout smoothie could provide that extra edge you're looking for.

If you're interested in the cognitive benefits of ashwagandha, such as enhanced focus and memory, consider combining it with brain-boosting foods. Including omega-3 rich foods like walnuts or fatty fish, along with ashwagandha, can foster a nutrient-rich diet that supports brain health and longevity.

Moreover, incorporating ashwagandha into your diet doesn't require an overhaul of your existing habits. Simple adjustments, like a morning brew or an evening supplement, make this adaptogen easily attainable. These small, manageable changes ensure you can maintain the habit and fully reap the long-term health benefits.

Lastly, always monitor any changes in your body or mood and adjust accordingly. Some individuals might experience mild side effects like digestive discomfort or drowsiness, especially when starting. Should these symptoms arise, adjusting the dosage or timing, and ensuring you're consuming it with food, can mitigate these issues.

Adding ashwagandha to your daily routine is a proactive step towards enhancing your overall well-being. Its versatility makes it an ideal candidate for inclusion in diverse culinary formats and supplementation methods. Whether you prefer a morning smoothie kick-start or a soothing evening tea, incorporating ashwagandha can pave the way for a balanced, healthful lifestyle.

Maca: Boosting Energy and Balance

Maca, often dubbed as "Peruvian ginseng," is a powerful adaptogen known for its remarkable ability to enhance energy, stamina, and overall balance. Native to the high altitudes of the Andes, this root vegetable has been used for centuries to combat fatigue and improve resilience against stress. Rich in essential amino acids, vitamins, and minerals, maca works to nourish the adrenal glands, promoting hormonal balance and fostering a sense of well-being. Incorporating maca into your daily regimen can be as simple as adding its powder form to smoothies, baked goods, or even morning coffee, making it an accessible superfood for those looking to experience its multifaceted benefits.

Maca-Enhanced Recipes tap into the potent benefits of this adaptogenic root, which has been utilized for centuries to boost energy, enhance mood, and balance hormones. As a superfood, maca offers a multitude of nutrients, including vitamins, minerals, and antioxidants. Its versatility in the kitchen makes it an exciting addition to a variety of recipes, from breakfast to dinner, and even snacks and desserts.

Maca powder can be easily integrated into your morning routine, starting with a *Maca-Infused Smoothie*. Blend a tablespoon of maca powder with a banana, a handful of spinach, a cup of almond milk, and a spoonful of almond butter. The result is a creamy and nutritious breakfast drink that energizes your day. The nutty, earthy flavor of maca pairs wonderfully with fruits and leafy greens, making it a seamless addition to any smoothie concoction.

For those who prefer a heartier start to their day, consider *Maca Oatmeal*. Simply add a teaspoon of maca powder to your cooked oats, along with some cinnamon, a dash of maple syrup, and perhaps a handful of berries or sliced banana. Maca not only adds a unique flavor but also enhances the nutritional profile of your oatmeal, providing sustained energy and a gentle mood boost throughout the morning.

If you're in the mood for baking, maca powder can elevate your favorite recipes with its nutritional benefits and distinctive taste. Try adding maca to your next batch of *Granola Bars*. Combine rolled oats, chopped nuts, dried fruits, a few tablespoons of honey, and a good sprinkle of maca powder. Press the mixture into a baking dish and bake until golden brown. These maca-infused bars make for a convenient, on-the-go snack that keeps you powered up between meals.

A unique way to incorporate maca into your diet is through savory recipes. For instance, add a tablespoon of maca powder to your *Mashed Sweet Potatoes* or even to the marinade for roasted vegetables. The subtle sweetness and earthy undertones of maca complement roasted root vegetables beautifully, offering a new twist on traditional dishes. This not only reinforces the nutritional quality of your meals but also introduces creative flavors to your palate.

Maca can also enhance salad dressings, providing a nutrient boost without overpowering the other ingredients. Whisk together olive oil, apple cider vinegar, a teaspoon of maca powder, Dijon mustard, and a touch of honey for a delicious and nutritious *Maca Vinaigrette*. Drizzle it over a mixed green salad or use it as a marinade for grilled chicken or tofu, adding both flavor and health benefits to your meal.

For dessert lovers, maca can be a delightful addition to various sweet treats. *Maca Chocolate Brownies* are an excellent example. Substitute a portion of the flour in your favorite brownie recipe with maca powder. The result is a richer, more nutrient-dense brownie with a slight caramel undertone. Not only does this provide an indulgent way to enjoy the benefits of maca, but it also satisfies your sweet tooth without compromising on health.

Maca Energy Balls are another fantastic way to enjoy this superfood. Blend dates, almonds, a tablespoon of maca powder, cocoa powder, and a pinch of sea salt in a food processor. Roll the mixture into small balls and refrigerate. These energy balls are perfect for a mid-afternoon pick-me-up or a post-workout snack, offering a balance of protein, healthy fats, and complex carbohydrates.

In beverages, maca shines as well. Stir a teaspoon of maca powder into your morning coffee or tea for an extra kick. Alternatively, a *Maca Latte* can be a soothing, warm beverage to start your day or unwind in the evening. Simply mix a cup of warm almond milk with a teaspoon of maca powder, a pinch of cinnamon, and a little honey or maple syrup to sweeten. Blend until frothy and enjoy a comforting, nutrient-rich drink.

For those who enjoy adventurous cooking, try incorporating maca into your sauces and soups. A *Maca-Infused Tomato Soup* can be both comforting and nourishing. Simply add a teaspoon of maca powder to your homemade or store-bought tomato soup, and blend well. The maca adds a subtle depth of flavor and boosts the soup's nutritional content, making it a heartier option for lunch or dinner.

Another savory option is to enhance your grain dishes with maca. For instance, in a *Maca Quinoa Pilaf*, cook quinoa as usual and stir in a teaspoon of maca powder along with your favorite herbs, vegetables, and a squeeze of lemon juice. This not only enriches the flavors but also transforms an everyday side dish into a super-nutritious meal component.

For a refreshing twist, maca can also be added to cold dishes such as *Fruit Salads*. Sprinkle a little maca powder over a mix of your favorite fruits, such as berries, kiwi, and citrus. Toss gently to combine. The natural sweetness and slight caramel flavor of maca complement the fruits wonderfully, making it a simple yet effective way to boost the nutritional profile of a light, refreshing dish.

No discussion of maca recipes would be complete without addressing its incorporation into healthier versions of traditional comfort foods. For instance, a *Maca-Enhanced Mac and Cheese* can transform this classic into a nutrient-packed meal. Prepare your cheese sauce as usual, then stir in a teaspoon of maca powder before mixing with the pasta. This adds a subtle, intriguing depth to the flavor while providing health benefits.

In addition to individual recipes, maca can be a handy addition to homemade snack mixes. Create a *Maca-Infused Trail Mix* by combining nuts, seeds, dried fruits, and a sprinkle of maca powder. This nutrient-dense snack mix is perfect for hiking, long workdays, or anytime you need a quick, healthy energy boost.

Maca's versatility extends even to beverages that can be enjoyed throughout the day. For instance, add a teaspoon of maca powder to your iced tea or lemonade. The slight earthiness of maca often complements the tartness of lemonade, resulting in a refreshing and vitalizing drink. Another option is a *Maca Mojito*, where you can mix maca powder with your traditional mojito ingredients. This cocktail becomes not only delicious but also unique and subtly nutritious, perfect for a summer gathering.

In conclusion, incorporating maca into your recipes is a straightforward and effective way to enhance your nutritional intake. Whether in smoothies, baked goods, savory dishes, or beverages, maca brings both flavor and health benefits to your table. The key is to experiment and find the combinations that best suit your taste and lifestyle, ensuring that you enjoy every step of your journey towards better health and longevity.

Chapter 13:
Sea Vegetables

Sea vegetables, often overlooked by many, are marvels of nutrition from the ocean that can dramatically enhance your health and longevity. These aquatic plants, such as nori and kelp, are packed with essential vitamins, minerals, and iodine, which are crucial for maintaining optimal thyroid function. Imagine the versatility of nori sheets, effortlessly transforming your lunches with sushi rolls or adding a crispy, salty punch to salads. Meanwhile, kelp brings its unique, umami-rich flavor to broths and stews, offering not just taste but a powerful dose of antioxidants. Incorporating these sea vegetables into your diet can be a game-changer, providing a potent blend of nutrients that can help detoxify the body, support cardiovascular health, and boost your overall vitality. Dive into the world of sea vegetables and unlock the secrets of the ocean for a healthier, more vibrant life.

Nori: The Superfood from the Sea

Nori, a type of edible seaweed popular in Japanese cuisine, is not only a delicious addition to dishes like sushi and salads but also packs a heavy nutritional punch. This sea vegetable is rich in essential nutrients such as iodine, which supports thyroid function, and vitamin B12, crucial for maintaining nerve health and producing red blood cells. High in protein and fiber while being low in calories, nori is an excellent choice for those who aim to maintain a healthy weight. Its high antioxidant content helps combat oxidative stress, contributing to overall longevity and wellness. Incorporating nori into your diet can be as simple as adding dried nori sheets to soups or using them as wraps for nutrient-dense snacks. The versatility and nutritional benefits of nori make it a superfood worth exploring.

Delicious Nori Recipes offer a gateway to harnessing the health-boosting benefits of this exceptional sea vegetable. Known primarily for its role in sushi, nori is versatile enough to enhance a myriad of dishes. Rich in vitamins A, B, and C, as well as iodine and iron, it packs a nutritional punch that can elevate your meal plans. Whether you're an accomplished chef or just venturing into the culinary world, integrating nori into your diet can be both easy and rewarding. Let's explore some creative and delectable ways to make nori a staple in your kitchen.

One of the simplest and most satisfying ways to enjoy nori is by making *Nori Chips*. These delightful snacks are not only easy to prepare but also offer a healthy alternative to traditional potato chips. To make nori chips, simply cut nori sheets into small squares or triangles, brush them lightly with olive oil, and sprinkle with sea salt. Arrange them on a baking sheet and bake at 300°F (150°C) for about 10 minutes or until they are crisp. You can customize the seasoning with a dash of garlic powder, paprika, or even nutritional yeast for an extra burst of flavor.

For those who enjoy a quicker snack, try *Homemade Nori Wraps*. Simply lay out a sheet of nori and fill it with your favorite vegetables, grains, and proteins. Ingredients like sliced avocado, shredded carrots, quinoa or brown rice, and even tofu work wonderfully in these wraps. Drizzle with a bit of soy sauce or a tangy tahini dressing, roll it up, and you have a nutritious, portable meal. These wraps are perfect for lunchboxes or a quick dinner solution.

If you're looking for a heartier meal option, *Nori-Wrapped Salmon* might just be the recipe for you. Start by preparing thin fillets of salmon, seasoning them lightly with salt, pepper, and a touch of lemon juice. Then, take nori sheets and wrap each salmon fillet snugly. You can secure the nori with a dab of water. Bake the wrapped fillets at 375°F (190°C) for about 20 minutes. The nori adds a unique flavor profile and an extra layer of nutrients to your meal. Serve with a side of steamed vegetables and a splash of tamari for a balanced, delicious dinner.

For a more exotic flavor, consider incorporating nori into a *Miso Nori Soup*. This soup combines the earthy flavors of miso with the oceanic taste of nori, creating a warming, nutrient-dense dish. Begin by boiling water and adding a couple of tablespoons of miso paste, stirring until it's dissolved. Add sliced shiitake mushrooms, tofu cubes, and a handful of thinly sliced nori strips. Let the soup simmer for about 10 minutes to allow the flavors to meld. Garnish with chopped green onions and enjoy a comforting bowl that's rich in umami and healthful goodness.

Nori-Infused Rice Bowls are another great way to incorporate this superfood into your meals. Start by cooking your favorite type of rice—white, brown, or even cauliflower rice if you're looking for a low-carb option. Once the rice is cooked, mix in crumbled pieces of nori sheets and a drizzle of sesame oil. Add a selection of toppings such as edamame, pickled ginger, cucumber slices, and a soft-boiled egg. This dish is not only visually appealing but also packed with diverse flavors and nutrients. It's perfect for a quick dinner or a filling lunch.

Don't forget about breakfast! Yes, you can even integrate nori into your morning routine with *Nori Avocado Toast*. Simply toast a slice of whole-grain bread, spread a generous amount of mashed avocado on top, and sprinkle with crumbled nori pieces. Add a squeeze of lemon juice and a pinch of sea salt to elevate the flavors. This quick and easy breakfast is not only delicious but also loaded with healthy fats, fiber, and the beneficial minerals found in nori.

For a flavorful side dish, try making *Nori-Seasoned Sweet Potato Fries*. Cut sweet potatoes into fry-sized wedges and toss them in olive oil. Spread them on a baking sheet and roast in the oven at 425°F (220°C) for about 25-30 minutes, turning them halfway through. Once they're crispy and golden, remove from the oven and toss with crumbled nori and a sprinkle of sesame seeds. These fries offer an exciting twist to a classic favorite, combining the sweetness of the potatoes with the savory umami of the nori.

If you're in the mood for something lighter, consider preparing a *Nori Seaweed Salad*. Combine rehydrated wakame seaweed (available in dried form at most health food stores) with thinly sliced cucumbers and carrots. Dress the salad with a mixture of rice vinegar, soy sauce, sesame oil, and a touch of honey or maple syrup. Sprinkle with toasted sesame seeds and crumbled pieces of nori. This refreshing salad is the perfect accompaniment to any main dish or a delightful snack on its own.

For a unique culinary adventure, why not make some *Nori Pesto*? This versatile sauce can be used on pasta, as a spread for sandwiches, or even as a dip for vegetables. In a food processor, blend together a handful of fresh basil, a few garlic cloves, a quarter cup of pine nuts, and a third cup of grated Parmesan cheese. Add a sheet of nori, torn into smaller pieces, and blend again. Gradually drizzle in olive oil until the mixture reaches a smooth, pesto-like consistency. The nori adds a subtle oceanic depth to the traditional pesto, making it a standout addition to your recipe repertoire.

Last but not least, don't overlook the simplicity of *Nori-Miso Dressing* for salads. To make this flavorful dressing, whisk together 2 tablespoons of white miso paste, 1 tablespoon of rice vinegar, 1 tablespoon of sesame oil, and 1 teaspoon of honey in a small bowl. Finely chop or crumble a sheet of nori and mix it into the dressing.

Drizzle over mixed greens or grain bowls for a rich umami flavor boost that will transform even the simplest salads into gourmet dishes.

Incorporating nori into your daily meals isn't just about boosting your health—it's also a way to bring a touch of creativity and global flair to your kitchen. From snacks to main courses to unique condiments, nori is a versatile superfood that seamlessly blends into various culinary styles while offering substantial health benefits. Enjoy experimenting with these **Delicious Nori Recipes** and discover new ways to elevate your everyday meals.

Kelp: A Hidden Gem

Kelp, often overshadowed by its flashier sea vegetable cousins, stands out as a powerhouse of nutrition waiting to be discovered. Rich in essential minerals like iodine, potassium, and magnesium, kelp supports thyroid function and cardiovascular health, playing a crucial role in maintaining overall well-being. It is incredibly versatile; you can add it to soups, salads, and even smoothies for a nutrient boost. What makes kelp particularly special is its ability to absorb and concentrate nutrients from the sea, providing a unique, low-calorie source of vitamins and antioxidants. Whether you're seeking to bolster your immune system or explore new culinary landscapes, incorporating this hidden gem into your diet can open the door to remarkable health benefits.

Ways to Include Kelp in Your Diet stands out as an underrated yet versatile ingredient that can be seamlessly woven into everyday meals, providing a nutrient boost and enhancing overall health. Packed with essential vitamins, minerals, and antioxidants, kelp is not just another sea vegetable; it's a powerhouse superfood. Integrating kelp into your diet doesn't have to be complicated. This section delves into easy and creative ways to make kelp a regular part of your culinary repertoire.

One of the simplest ways to include kelp in your diet is by using kelp granules or flakes. These can be effortlessly sprinkled over salads, soups, or even popcorn. Kelp granules often come in shaker bottles, making it convenient to add a dash of nutrition to almost any dish. The mildly salty taste of granules can replace traditional table salt, offering a healthier alternative rich in iodine and other trace minerals.

For those who enjoy making smoothies, adding a spoonful of kelp powder to your favorite blend is an excellent option. The powder form of kelp integrates well with fruits and vegetables, masking any oceanic flavor while still delivering its nutritional benefits. Smoothies are great because you can customize them based on your taste while ensuring that you're getting a good dose of essential nutrients.

Another great way to incorporate kelp is in soups and stews. Kelp's umami flavor enhances these dishes without overpowering other ingredients. Try adding dried kelp strips (also known as kombu) to broths or stock. Not only does kelp enrich the flavor profile, but it also adds essential vitamins like A, C, and E, and minerals such as calcium and magnesium. Kombu is a popular ingredient in Japanese cuisine used to create dashi, a foundational broth used in numerous dishes.

Kelp noodles are a gluten-free, low-carb alternative to traditional pasta. These translucent, slightly-crunchy noodles are made from kelp's inner core and can be found in most health food stores. They don't need to be boiled; simply rinse and add them to your favorite pasta sauces, salads, or stir-fries. The neutral taste of kelp noodles allows them to absorb the flavors of whatever dish you're preparing, making them incredibly versatile.

Incorporating kelp into your diet can also be as simple as snacking on kelp snacks or chips. These are often baked and seasoned, providing a crunchy, savory snack that's much healthier than traditional potato chips. Kelp snacks are typically available in various flavors, so you can experiment to find your favorite.

For a traditional approach, consider making kelp salad. Wakame, a type of kelp, is commonly used in seaweed salads. Simply soak dried wakame in water until it rehydrates, then toss it with sesame oil, vinegar, soy sauce, and sesame seeds. This salad pairs well with sushi, grilled fish, or can be enjoyed on its own. It's a tasty and refreshing way to get your daily dose of sea vegetables.

Taking a more culinary approach, you can integrate kelp into homemade sushi rolls. Nori, another type of sea vegetable, is widely known for its role in wrapping sushi rolls. However, including a thin strip of kelp along with fish, vegetables, and rice within the roll adds another layer of nutrition and texture. It's a subtle yet effective way to enhance your sushi game.

Kelp can be used as a base in fermented foods such as kimchi. Adding kelp to your kimchi not only diversifies the nutrient content but also improves gut health through increased probiotic action. The natural fermentation process of kimchi enhances the bioavailability of kelp's nutrients, making them easier for your body to absorb.

Experimentation is key when working kelp into your diet. You could create kelp-infused dressings and marinades to elevate the nutrient profile of your meals. Blend kelp powder with olive oil, lemon juice, garlic, and a touch of honey for a nutrient-dense salad dressing. Or, create a marinade for fish or tofu using soy sauce, ginger, garlic, and finely chopped kelp. These small additions can make a big difference in flavor and health benefits.

Interestingly, kelp can also be used in baking. Incorporating kelp powder into bread or cracker recipes can enrich the nutritional value of these baked goods without altering the taste significantly. A teaspoon of kelp powder added to your next batch of homemade bread can provide a subtle health boost without overpowering other flavors.

For a sweet take, try making energy balls or protein bars incorporating kelp. Mix dates, nuts, seeds, and a small amount of kelp powder in a food processor, roll them into bite-sized balls, and refrigerate. These energy balls offer a quick, nutrient-packed snack that combines the health benefits of kelp with the protein and energy boost from nuts and seeds.

Another user-friendly option is to look for kelp supplements available in pill or capsule form. While whole food sources are often preferred for nutrient intake, supplements can be beneficial for those with dietary restrictions or for added convenience. Always consult with a healthcare professional before adding any new supplements to your routine.

Adding kelp to your diet isn't just about the nutritional benefits; it's also about cultivating a broader palate and experimenting with new flavors and textures. The versatility of kelp makes it easy to sneak into almost any meal, turning ordinary dishes into superfood feats. As you continue to explore and integrate different superfoods, kelp offers a simple yet powerful way to enhance your diet, contribute to your health, and support longevity.

Chapter 14:
Citrus Fruits

Citrus fruits stand out as vibrant, juicy powerhouses packed with essential nutrients that benefit our health in myriad ways. Oranges, often hailed as the quintessential source of vitamin C, bolster our immune system and fend off ailments. Lemons, on the other hand, offer unparalleled detoxifying properties, making them a staple in cleanses and morning rituals alike. The tangy zest and refreshing juice of these fruits not only elevate culinary creations but also provide antioxidants, fiber, and a medley of other vitamins and minerals that support overall wellness. Incorporating citrus fruits into your daily diet can brighten dishes and enhance flavors, all while promoting longevity and vitality. So, next time you enjoy a slice of orange or a squeeze of lemon, remember you're making a delicious step towards better health.

Oranges: Vitamin C Powerhouses

Oranges are a standout among citrus fruits, beloved not only for their juicy sweetness but also for their impressive Vitamin C content. One medium-sized orange can provide over 100% of the daily recommended intake of Vitamin C, making them a key player in boosting your immune system, enhancing skin health, and aiding in the absorption of iron from plant-based foods. This nutrient-dense fruit also offers other essential vitamins and minerals such as potassium, folate, and antioxidants like flavonoids, which help combat oxidative stress and inflammation. Incorporating oranges into your daily diet, whether through fresh slices, juice, or zest in recipes, is a delicious and effective way to enhance your overall health and longevity.

Recipes Featuring Oranges are a celebration of nature's bountiful gifts. Not only are oranges incredibly versatile, but they're also brimming with nutrients that can give your health a significant boost. Known for their high vitamin C content, oranges can be the perfect ingredient to incorporate into everyday meals for a citrusy kick and a healthful twist. Whether you're whipping up a quick breakfast, a hearty salad, or a decadent dessert, there's always room for oranges in your cuisine.

Kickstart your day with an invigorating *Orange and Avocado Smoothie*. This refreshing blend is perfect for a morning pick-me-up. Combine freshly squeezed orange juice with ripe avocado, a handful of spinach, and a touch of honey. Blend until smooth and frothy. The avocado renders a creamy texture while the orange juice adds a tangy zest. Spinach offers a boost of iron and fiber, making this smoothie not only delicious but also nutrient-dense.

For a mid-morning snack, try an *Orange and Almond Granola*. Combine rolled oats, sliced almonds, orange zest, and a hint of cinnamon. Drizzle with honey and a bit of melted coconut oil before baking until golden brown. The orange zest imparts a marvelous citrus aroma and flavor, complementing the nutty crunch of the almonds. This granola can be served over yogurt or enjoyed on its own as a crunchy snack.

Moving on to lunch, consider a vibrant *Orange and Beet Salad*. Start with roasted beets, which add an earthy sweetness, and mix them with orange segments, thinly sliced red onions, and a sprinkle of goat cheese. Dress it all in a simple vinaigrette made of olive oil, vinegar, orange juice, and a touch of mustard. This salad is not only a feast for the eyes with its brilliant colors but also a powerhouse of antioxidants, perfect for boosting your immune system.

If you're craving something more savory, an *Orange-Glazed Tofu Stir-Fry* might be just the ticket. Start by pressing and cubing tofu, then marinate it in a mixture of fresh orange juice, soy sauce, garlic, and ginger. Stir-fry with an array of colorful bell peppers and snap peas before adding the marinade as a glaze in the final minutes of cooking. The bright, citrusy glaze complements the savory undertones of the soy sauce, creating a dish that's both flavorful and rich in plant-based protein.

For a family dinner, an *Orange and Herb Roasted Chicken* is a surefire hit. Begin by stuffing a whole chicken with a few orange halves, garlic cloves, and fresh rosemary. Rub the outside with olive oil, salt, pepper, and additional orange zest before roasting it to perfection. The golden, crispy skin with a hint of citrus pairs wonderfully with the aromatic herbs, making it a satisfying and elegant main course.

No meal is complete without a touch of sweetness, and an *Orange-Infused Dark Chocolate Mousse* can be the perfect finale. Melt high-quality dark chocolate and fold it gently into whipped cream with a splash of orange liqueur and a pinch of orange zest. Allow it to set in individual serving bowls and garnish with a candied orange peel. The deep, rich flavor of the chocolate, enhanced by the bright citrus notes, provides a decadent and satisfying dessert that remains surprisingly light.

Even your beverages can benefit from the inclusion of oranges. A *Spiced Orange Tea* can be the perfect conclusion to a day. Brew your favorite black tea and add in freshly squeezed orange juice, a stick of cinnamon, and a few cloves. Simmer for a few minutes to let the spices infuse, then strain and serve hot. The warmth of the spices paired with the refreshing citrus creates a comforting and immune-boosting drink, ideal for unwinding.

For those looking to experiment further, consider making a *Homemade Orange Marmalade*. This spread can elevate your breakfast toast to gourmet status. Combine thinly sliced oranges, including the peel, with sugar and water. Simmer until the mixture thickens and reaches the perfect consistency. The result is a sweet, slightly tart marmalade that captures the essence of fresh oranges. It pairs well not only with bread but also as a glaze for meats or a topping for desserts.

Visually stunning and flavor-packed, an *Orange and Pistachio Couscous* can be a delightful side dish or light main course. Prepare couscous according to package instructions and toss with orange segments, chopped pistachios, finely chopped mint, and a drizzle of olive oil. Finish with a squeeze of fresh orange juice. The nuttiness of the pistachios juxtaposed with the citrusy burst of the oranges and the freshness of mint creates a harmonious and delightful dish.

The possibilities with oranges in the kitchen are truly endless. They can brighten a savory dish, add a sweet and tangy note to desserts, or simply provide a refreshing element to your beverages. With a little creativity and a keen understanding of flavors, oranges can be seamlessly integrated into your daily meals, helping you to reap the numerous health benefits they offer while tantalizing your taste buds.

Lemons: Detoxifiers

Incorporating lemons into your daily diet is a simple yet powerful way to enhance your body's natural detoxification processes. Rich in vitamin C and antioxidants, lemons help to neutralize free radicals and reduce inflammation. They also promote digestion and hydration, which are essential for flushing out toxins. Squeeze fresh lemon juice into your water, add it to salads, or use it in marinades to reap these benefits. By making lemons a staple in your nutritional regimen, you can support your liver, the body's main detox organ, and keep your body running smoothly.

Using Lemons Daily is one of the simplest and most effective steps you can take to enhance your health and longevity. This citrus gem, renowned for its detoxifying properties, offers more than just a zesty flavor; it's a nutritional powerhouse that can easily be incorporated into your daily routine. From morning rituals to evening meals, here's how you can make lemons an indispensable part of your daily life.

Kickstart your day with a glass of warm lemon water. The fresh lemon juice helps stimulate your digestive system and flush out toxins accumulated overnight. To prepare, simply squeeze half a lemon into a glass of warm water. You might be tempted to add sweeteners, but resist; the natural tartness of lemon is invigorating on its own. This daily habit supports liver function, improves digestion, and boosts your immune system due to its high vitamin C content.

Moving on to breakfast, lemons can brighten up many morning meals. Think of a squeeze of lemon juice over avocado toast or oatmeal. If you're a fan of smoothies, lemon juice can be an excellent addition. It not only enhances flavor but also increases the absorption of iron from the greens in the smoothie. For an extra nutritional boost, add in a teaspoon of chia seeds along with a few drops of fresh lemon juice.

Lunchtime offers more opportunities for incorporating lemons. A simple lemon vinaigrette can elevate any salad. To make it, whisk together fresh lemon juice, olive oil, a touch of Dijon mustard, and a pinch of salt and pepper. This light and tangy dressing pairs well with mixed greens, quinoa salads, or even grilled chicken. Another tip: lemon wedges are a perfect addition to your water bottle, making hydration a flavorful experience.

An afternoon snack can also benefit from the zest of lemons. Try making lemon hummus. Blend chickpeas, tahini, garlic, olive oil, and a generous squeeze of lemon juice until smooth. This can be paired with a variety of veggies or whole-grain crackers. The lemon juice not only adds refreshing acidity but also helps break down the beans, making the hummus easier to digest.

Dinner time is where lemons can truly shine. Marinating proteins in lemon juice can tenderize meat and infuse it with a subtle citrus flavor. A classic example is a lemon and herb marinade for fish or chicken. Mix lemon juice, olive oil, minced garlic, and a handful of fresh herbs like rosemary or thyme. Let your protein of choice marinate for at least an hour before cooking. The result is a moist, flavorful dish with a hint of brightness from the lemon.

Don't forget about side dishes. A squeeze of lemon can enhance the flavor of steamed or roasted vegetables, such as broccoli, asparagus, or zucchini. For a simple yet delicious side, toss roasted veggies with lemon juice and zest right before serving. This can elevate the natural sweetness of the vegetables and add a refreshing contrast.

Lemons also play a starring role in numerous desserts without tipping the scale on sugar content. A favorite is a lemon-infused Greek yogurt. By mixing fresh lemon juice and zest into plain Greek yogurt and drizzling a bit of honey, you create a light, tangy, and nutritious treat. If you enjoy baking, consider lemon bars made with almond flour for a gluten-free option. These bars can be sweetened with natural sweeteners like maple syrup or agave for a healthier take on a classic dessert.

Beyond the kitchen, lemons offer various practical uses in daily life. Their natural antibacterial and antiviral properties make them excellent in homemade cleaning solutions. Mix lemon juice with water and a bit of white vinegar for an effective surface cleaner. Additionally, the aroma of lemon has been shown to boost mood and increase energy levels, making it a perfect ingredient for natural air fresheners. Simply simmer lemon slices with herbs like rosemary or lavender on the stove for a fragrant, uplifting scent.

Don't forget that using lemons daily can also have positive effects on your skin. The vitamin C in lemons is a potent antioxidant that can help protect your skin from damage caused by free radicals. For an easy at-home facial treatment, mix lemon juice with honey and apply it to your face. Leave it on for about 10-15 minutes before rinsing. This simple mask can help brighten your complexion and reduce the appearance of blemishes.

Additionally, lemons can be a great aid in weight management. Pectin fiber is found in the pulp of the lemon and can help reduce hunger cravings. To take advantage of this, consume the whole lemon, not just the juice. You can blend the entire fruit, including the peel, into smoothies or use thin slices in teas and salads.

At the end of the day, winding down with a cup of warm lemon and ginger tea can be soothing and beneficial. This simple tonic can aid digestion and provide a calming effect. To make, boil water and add a few slices of ginger and half a lemon. Let it steep for a few minutes, and sweeten with a touch of honey if desired.

By consistently incorporating lemons into your daily regimen, you harness their full spectrum of health benefits. Whether through beverages, meals, or even skincare, the versatility of lemons ensures you'll never run out of ways to use this superfood. Experiment with different recipes and methods to find what works best for you, and enjoy the zest and vitality lemons bring to your life.

Chapter 15:
High-Quality Proteins

When it comes to fostering the ideal foundation for longevity and vibrant health, high-quality proteins play an indispensable role within our diet. Their contributions extend beyond mere muscle repair—these proteins are integral for hormonal balance, enzyme function, and even immune system fortification. By incorporating nutrient-dense sources such as wild-caught salmon, which is brimming with omega-3 fatty acids, and pastured eggs, often hailed as nature's multivitamin, one can significantly enhance their overall nutrient profile. These proteins not only supply the essential amino acids our bodies can't produce on their own but also offer additional health benefits. For instance, the anti-inflammatory properties of omega-3s in salmon support heart health, while eggs provide a wealth of vitamins and minerals like vitamin D and choline. Prioritizing these high-quality protein sources can bring about improved energy levels, sharper cognitive functions, and a robust defense against chronic diseases, setting the stage for a healthier, longer life.

Salmon: The Omega-3 Rich Protein

Salmon stands out as a high-quality protein, celebrated for its rich content of omega-3 fatty acids, which play a crucial role in promoting cardiovascular health, reducing inflammation, and supporting brain function. By incorporating salmon into your regular diet, you're not only enjoying a versatile and delicious seafood option, but you're also ensuring a robust intake of essential nutrients such as vitamins D and B12, selenium, and various antioxidants. Wild-caught salmon is often recommended due to its lower contaminant levels and higher nutrient profile compared to its farmed counterpart. Whether you prefer it grilled, baked, or even raw in sushi, making salmon a staple in your meal planning can be a flavorful and smart choice for long-term health and vitality.

Cooking Tips for Salmon One of the most versatile and nutrient-dense proteins around, salmon is a superstar in the world of superfoods, especially for those looking to enhance their health and longevity. The anti-inflammatory omega-3 fatty acids found in salmon are well-documented for their cardiovascular benefits. However, preparing and cooking salmon can be tricky if you're not familiar with its unique qualities. Here, we'll dive into some essential tips for cooking salmon in ways that preserve its nutrients, enhance its flavors, and suit various culinary preferences.

First and foremost, selecting the right type of salmon is key. Wild-caught varieties like Sockeye, Coho, and King salmon are usually richer in nutrients compared to their farmed counterparts. They're lower in environmental contaminants and higher in omega-3 fatty acids. When purchasing salmon, look for firm flesh and a fresh, oceanic scent. The color should be vibrant—ranging from bright pink to deep red, depending on the species. Avoid fillets with brown or gray spots, as these are signs of oxidation and age.

Once you've selected your salmon, it's important to decide on the cooking method that best suits both your taste preferences and nutritional goals. One popular way to cook salmon is by grilling. Grilling can add a smoky flavor that elevates the fish without requiring excessive oils or other fats. To prevent the salmon from sticking to the grill, use a brush to apply a light coating of olive oil on the fish and the grill grates. Marinating the salmon for about 15-30 minutes beforehand can also enhance its flavor profile. Avoid over-marinating, as acidic ingredients like lemon or vinegar can break down the fish.

Another effective method is baking. Baking salmon is a straightforward way to ensure even cooking while retaining moisture. Preheat your oven to 400°F (200°C). Lay the salmon on a baking sheet lined with parchment paper or aluminum foil for easy cleanup. Season with herbs like dill and thyme, and a sprinkle of sea salt. You can also add a squeeze of lemon for brightness. Bake for about 12-15 minutes, depending on the thickness of the fillet—when the salmon flakes easily with a fork, it's done.

If you're after something even richer, consider pan-searing. This method results in a crispy exterior while keeping the inside tender and juicy. Heat a tablespoon of healthy oil (like avocado or olive oil) in a non-stick skillet over medium-high heat. Pat the salmon dry to ensure a good sear, then place it skin-side up in the pan. Sear for about 4-6 minutes on each side, depending on the fillet's thickness. For an added layer of flavor, finish with a pat of grass-fed butter and a garlic clove during the last minute of cooking.

For those looking to keep things light and nutrient-rich, poaching is an excellent option. Poaching preserves the delicate flavors of the salmon without adding any extra fat. Fill a deep skillet with about an inch of water, wine, or broth, and add aromatics like bay leaves, peppercorns, and a slice of lemon. Bring to a boil and reduce to a simmer, then gently place the salmon in the liquid. Cook for about 10 minutes or until the salmon is opaque throughout.

If you're in a hurry but still want a nutritious meal, broiling is your best friend. This high-heat method cooks salmon quickly, making it ideal for weeknight dinners. Preheat your broiler and position an oven rack about six inches from the heat source. Place the salmon on a broiling pan or a baking sheet lined with aluminum foil. Season to taste, and broil for about 7-10 minutes, depending on the thickness. A well-broiled piece of salmon should have a lightly browned top and a flaky interior.

Looking for a more nuanced flavor? Try sous-vide cooking. This method involves sealing the salmon in a vacuum bag and cooking it in a water bath at a precisely controlled temperature. Sous-vide offers unparalleled moisture retention and texture. Heat your water bath to about 120°F (49°C) for a softer, sashimi-like texture or 130°F (54°C) for a firmer, flaky texture. It generally takes around 30 minutes, and you can finish the salmon with a quick sear in a hot pan for extra flavor.

Ultimately, the best way to cook salmon depends on your preference and lifestyle. If you're more traditional, you might enjoy methods like grilling and baking. For those into modern cooking techniques, sous-vide and broiling offer exciting alternatives. Whichever method you choose, the key to perfect salmon lies in not overcooking it. Overcooked salmon can become dry and lose its rich flavor and nutritional benefits.

To further boost the nutritional value of your salmon dish, consider the sides and garnishes you pair with it. Vegetables like asparagus, Brussels sprouts, and spinach complement salmon's richness and contribute essential vitamins and minerals. Preparing these sides simply by roasting or steaming helps preserve their nutritional value. You can also serve the salmon with a quinoa salad or a bed of whole grain rice to make a balanced, nutrient-dense meal.

When it comes to seasoning, don't underestimate the power of simplicity. A squeeze of fresh lemon and a sprinkle of sea salt bring out salmon's natural flavors without overpowering them. Fresh herbs like dill, parsley, and chives add brightness, while ground pepper and paprika offer a subtle kick. For those who enjoy a bit of complexity, a homemade glaze of honey, mustard, and a dash of soy sauce can provide a delightful contrast of flavors.

For a more global culinary experience, consider experimenting with different spice blends and marinades. A miso-marinated salmon brings a taste of Japan to your table, while a Cajun blackened seasoning offers a robust, southern flair. Mediterranean-style combinations using olive oil, lemon, garlic, and oregano can transport you straight to a sunnier locale. The possibilities are endless, and experimenting with different flavors and techniques can make cooking salmon a fulfilling endeavor.

In summary, cooking salmon doesn't have to be an intimidating task. With a few simple tips and techniques, you can prepare delicious and healthful salmon dishes that will keep you coming back for more. Remember, the key is to start with quality ingredients and avoid overcooking to retain all those wonderful nutrients. Armed with these cooking tips, you're well on your way to mastering salmon and incorporating this omega-3 rich superfood into your dietary routine for better health and longevity.

Eggs: Nature's Multivitamin

When it comes to high-quality proteins, eggs stand out as an extraordinarily efficient source, earning their title as nature's multivitamin. Packed with essential amino acids, vitamins, and minerals, eggs provide not just protein but an array of nutrients that support muscle growth, brain function, and overall vitality. Each egg is a compact powerhouse, containing Vitamin B12, riboflavin, and selenium, along with important antioxidants like lutein and zeaxanthin, which promote eye health. Including eggs in your diet is a simple, versatile way to boost your intake of critical nutrients, all within a low-calorie package. Whether you prefer them scrambled, poached, or boiled, incorporating eggs into your meals can make a significant impact on your health and longevity.

Versatile Egg Recipes highlight just how adaptable and beneficial the simple egg can be in your daily diet. Whether you're looking to load up on protein, pack in some essential vitamins and minerals, or simply enjoy a delicious meal, eggs are a fantastic choice. They're rich in vitamin B12, riboflavin, and selenium, making them a nutritional powerhouse that's hard to beat. With a high protein content, they're great for muscle repair and satiety. Their versatility makes them an excellent component in any meal plan focused on enhancing health and longevity

Starting your day with a hearty egg breakfast can set the tone for a productive and energetic day. Consider the classic vegetable omelet. Whip up three eggs, add a splash of milk, and generously fill it with spinach, tomatoes, and bell peppers. A sprinkling of cheese can increase the dish's calcium content. The beauty of an omelet is its flexibility–swap out vegetables based on your preference or what's in season. High in protein and bursting with fiber from the vegetables, it's a meal that can keep you full for hours.

For a breakfast option that's a little different, try making a batch of egg muffins. Beat a dozen eggs and mix them with diced vegetables, cooked quinoa, and shredded cheese. Pour the mixture into a greased muffin tin and bake. These muffins can be made ahead of time and stored in the refrigerator for quick morning meals. This recipe is not only nutritious but also practical for those with a busy lifestyle. These small, portable breakfast bites offer a balanced combination of proteins and veggies, making them perfect for on-the-go nutrition.

While breakfast might be the most obvious time for eggs, don't limit their consumption to the morning hours. A classic egg salad can make a nutrient-dense lunch. Built on a base of boiled eggs, a light touch of Greek yogurt or avocado can replace traditional mayonnaise, adding a creamy texture without the saturated fat. Herbs like dill and chives, along with a bit of mustard, can elevate the flavor profile. Serve it on a bed of leafy greens or whole grain bread for a well-rounded, satisfying midday meal.

Want something even more filling? Shakshuka, a Middle Eastern dish of poached eggs in a spicy tomato sauce, is an excellent option for lunch or dinner. The dish starts with a rich, spiced tomato base made by simmering onions, bell peppers, and tomatoes with a blend of spices like paprika and cumin. Eggs are then gently cracked into the sauce and allowed to poach until just set. This dish, which can be served with whole grain bread or pita, offers a delightful mix of textures and a significant nutrient boost thanks to the tomatoes and peppers.

Eggs play a starring role in many culinary traditions around the world, providing ample opportunity to explore global flavors while prioritizing your health. Asian cuisine, for example, features egg drop soup, a straightforward yet delicious soup that combines beaten eggs, chicken broth, and green onions. This soup is light yet satisfying, perfect for a warm appetizer or a light meal. By incorporating bone broth into the recipe, you can boost the soup's nutritional profile significantly.

For a more substantial dinner, consider quiche. Although it has a reputation for being rich and calorie-dense, it's easy to lighten up with the right ingredients. A crustless quiche can cut down on unnecessary carbs and fats. Incorporate ingredients like smoked salmon, a known superfood rich in omega-3 fatty acids, spinach, and a mix of cheeses for a dish brimming with flavor and nutrients. This versatile dish can be enjoyed warm or at room temperature, making it ideal for meal prep.

Speaking of meal prep, don't forget the role of eggs in simple yet effective snacks. Hard-boiled eggs are a convenient, protein-packed snack that can be jazzed up with a dash of salt or a sprinkle of paprika. Another snack idea is deviled eggs, which can be made healthier by replacing some or all of the mayonnaise with Greek yogurt. Add mustard and your choice of herbs for an additional nutrient boost.

These make excellent appetizers for gatherings or a satisfying bite between meals.

Beyond typical savory applications, eggs also work wonders in baked goods when you're looking for a healthier sweet treat. Consider swapping conventional desserts for nutrient-packed options like an avocado chocolate mousse, which uses eggs as a key component to achieve a silky-smooth finish. By combining ripe avocados, raw cacao, a bit of honey, and eggs, you get a dessert rich in healthy fats, antioxidants, and essential nutrients. This mousse offers a guilt-free way to satisfy your sweet tooth while simultaneously boosting your intake of superfoods.

An often-overlooked advantage of eggs is their role in creating emulsions, which can be used to craft nutritious sauces and dressings. A homemade mayonnaise, for instance, can be made with egg yolks, a healthy oil like avocado or olive oil, and a splash of lemon juice. Unlike store-bought versions, which can contain unhealthy fats and additives, homemade mayo crafted from quality ingredients can offer a burst of natural, wholesome flavors while supporting a nutrient-rich diet.

For those with a taste for adventure, explore incorporating eggs into Asian-inspired bowls. A soft-boiled egg perched atop a bed of quinoa, edamame, shredded carrots, and cabbage with a drizzle of tamari sauce creates a nutrient-dense meal. This type of bowl, commonly referred to as a "Buddha bowl," can be customized endlessly to include a variety of superfoods. Eggs provide the protein punch, complementing the vitamins and minerals found within the rest of the ingredients.

The versatility of eggs is not just limited to meals and snacks; they also shine in drinks. Eggnog is a traditional holiday beverage that can be enhanced with the addition of superfoods like turmeric for added anti-inflammatory properties. By using raw eggs sourced from reputable suppliers, honey or maple syrup for sweetness, and a plant-based milk, you can enjoy a wholesome version of this festive drink. Incorporating ingredients like nutmeg or cinnamon provides additional antioxidant benefits.

If you've never considered using eggs in savory pancake recipes, now's the time. Combining eggs with ingredients like flaxseed meal and spinach produces a batter that's loaded with fiber, omega-3 fatty acids, and essential vitamins. These savory pancakes can be enjoyed with a topping of avocado or a sprinkle of feta cheese, offering a novel, nutritious twist on a beloved breakfast food. This recipe also serves as a fantastic way to sneak more greens into your diet.

Often, the simplest methods for preparing eggs are the best. A perfectly scrambled egg, when cooked gently and seasoned well, is a delight. By cooking the eggs slowly over low heat and stirring constantly, you achieve a creamy texture that feels indulgent yet is incredibly healthy. Adding superfoods like finely chopped kale or turmeric can enhance both the nutritional value and the flavor. Serve atop a slice of whole grain or sourdough toast to complete this quick, healthy meal.

In closing, exploring the versatile world of egg recipes is a gratifying journey. Eggs' adaptability and nutrient density make them an unbeatable ingredient in

Chapter 16:
Superfood Beverages

From invigorating green tea to nutrient-packed smoothies, superfood beverages are a seamless way to incorporate a variety of essential nutrients into your day. Green tea, renowned for its high antioxidant content, offers not just a gentle pick-me-up, but also support for heart health and metabolism. Smoothies provide a versatile canvas to blend fruits, vegetables, nuts, and even adaptogens, creating delicious and nutrient-dense drinks tailored to your specific health needs. Whether you are looking to boost your immune system, increase energy levels, or simply enjoy a refreshing drink, these superfood beverages are your ticket to enhanced vitality and longevity.

Green Tea: Antioxidant Elixir

Green tea has long been revered as a potent source of antioxidants, offering a multitude of health benefits that extend far beyond its soothing taste. Rich in polyphenols, particularly catechins like EGCG, this ancient beverage fights oxidative stress and inflammation, potentially reducing the risk of chronic diseases such as heart disease and cancer. Beyond its well-documented health properties, green tea also supports cognitive function and metabolic health. Incorporating green tea into daily life is simple; from a traditional hot brew to incorporating its powdered form, matcha, in smoothies and baked goods, the versatile applications make it effortless to harness its healing properties. Introduce green tea into your routine, and relish its role in promoting longevity and well-being.

How to Enjoy Green Tea is a discovery of flavor, heritage, and health benefits that align seamlessly with the goal of enhancing one's well-being through superfoods. Green tea, unparalleled in its historical significance and modern acclaim, can be enjoyed in numerous ways to suit diverse palates and lifestyles.

Getting the most out of green tea starts with understanding the variety it offers. Traditional green teas like Sencha and Matcha bring different experiences to the table. Sencha, a quintessential Japanese green tea, is typically enjoyed as an everyday drink due to its light, refreshing flavor. Matcha, on the other hand, is finely ground green tea powder that delivers a full-bodied, vegetal taste and is often celebrated for its ceremonial roots in Japanese culture.

Preparation is key to enjoying the perfect cup of green tea. A common mistake is using boiling water, which can scorch the delicate leaves and produce bitterness. Instead, allow boiled water to cool slightly, aiming for a temperature around 160-170°F (70-80°C). Steeping time matters too; for Sencha, 1-2 minutes is ideal, while Matcha is whisked vigorously in water until frothy. Experiment with steeping times to find your preferred strength.

Another way to savor green tea is by incorporating it into recipes. Matcha lattes have surged in popularity, blending the antioxidant-rich powder with steamed milk (or a plant-based alternative) for a creamy, energizing drink. For a refreshing twist, try an iced green tea infused with mint and lemon – a perfect blend for hot summer days. Culinary uses of green tea extend to baking, where Matcha's vibrant green color and unique flavor can enhance cakes, cookies, and even savory dishes like matcha soba noodles.

Pairing green tea with food can elevate both the tea and the meal. Sencha pairs well with light, savory foods such as sushi and salads due to its clean and grassy notes. Matcha, with its more robust flavor, complements sweet desserts like mochi and dark chocolate. When hosting a tea tasting, consider a progression from lighter green teas to more intense varieties, allowing each tea's nuanced flavors to shine.

Health benefits amplify the experience of enjoying green tea. Rich in catechins, particularly EGCG (epigallocatechin gallate), green tea has been shown to boost metabolism, improve brain function, and contribute to heart health. Including green tea in your daily routine can be as simple as substituting it for less healthy beverages. Start your morning with a cup of green tea instead of coffee, enjoy it in the afternoon for a gentle energy boost, or create a calming evening ritual with a warm cup after dinner.

Mindfulness plays a significant role in the enjoyment of green tea. The preparation and sipping process can be a meditative practice, allowing for a moment of tranquility in a busy day. Focus on the aroma, flavor, and warmth of each sip. This mindful approach not only enhances the sensory experience but also fosters a deeper appreciation for the ancient traditions and modern health benefits that green tea embodies.

Adventurous tea drinkers may explore blending green tea with other superfoods to create powerhouse beverages. Add a dash of turmeric and a sprinkle of black pepper to a cup of green tea for an anti-inflammatory boost. Alternatively, combine green tea with fresh ginger and honey for a soothing, immune-supportive drink.

If you're new to green tea, start with a quality green tea from a reputable source to ensure you're getting the full spectrum of benefits and flavors. As you become more familiar with the taste, explore different types and preparations. Green tea is a versatile and adaptable superfood that can easily become a staple in your wellness routine.

Travel enthusiasts and those interested in cultural experiences might appreciate exploring the traditional tea ceremonies of Japan. Participating in a tea ceremony or learning the intricate steps of Matcha preparation can provide a deeper connection to the cultural significance of green tea, enriching your enjoyment and understanding of this venerable beverage.

Incorporating green tea into a balanced diet is straightforward and rewarding. Alongside other nutrient-dense superfoods, green tea can help you maintain optimal health and vitality. Regular consumption has been linked to numerous health benefits, from reducing the risk of chronic diseases to enhancing cognitive functions. By making green tea a part of your daily habit, you're not just enjoying a flavorful drink; you're investing in your long-term health.

Whether you savor it hot or cold, whisked in a bowl or steeped in a cup, green tea offers a harmonious blend of flavor and wellness benefits. Its versatility makes it easy to integrate into any lifestyle, providing a simple yet profound way to enhance your diet with a superfood that has stood the test of time.

To conclude, the journey of discovering how to enjoy green tea is both personal and transformative. From its traditional roots to modern-day innovations, green tea continues to be an essential part of a healthy, superfood-rich diet. Explore various types and preparation methods, pair your teas thoughtfully with meals, and incorporate mindfulness into your tea rituals. In doing so, you'll not only savor a world of flavors but also harness one of nature's most potent superfoods for enhancing your health and longevity.

Smoothies: Nutrient-Packed Drinks

Jump into the delightful world of smoothies, where nutrition meets convenience in a deliciously vibrant fusion. These nutrient-packed drinks are your gateway to effortlessly incorporating a myriad of superfoods into your diet, all while tantalizing your taste buds. Imagine blending antioxidant-rich berries, leafy greens, and healthy fats from nuts and seeds, creating a powerhouse beverage ready to kickstart your day or recharge your afternoon. Not only are smoothies quick to prepare, but they're also incredibly versatile—tailor them to your specific health needs by adding protein, fiber, or adaptogens. Whether you're battling a hectic schedule or simply craving something nutritious and refreshing, smoothies offer a seamless blend of flavor and health benefits, empowering you to make every sip count.

Crafting Perfect Smoothie Blends offers a unique opportunity to incorporate a vast array of superfoods into a single, delicious drink. Smoothies are versatile and can be tailored to meet your nutritional needs, making them an excellent vehicle for enhancing health and longevity. They're quick to prepare, easy to consume, and an efficient way to pack multiple nutrient-dense ingredients into your diet.

Whether you're new to blending or a seasoned pro, understanding the basic components of a perfect smoothie can make all the difference. Smoothies generally consist of four main parts: a liquid base, fruits or vegetables, a protein source, and additional superfood boosters for extra nutrition. Let's delve into each category to help you create balanced and delectable blends.

First up, the liquid base. This forms the foundation of your smoothie, dictating its fluidity and overall texture. Common choices include water, nut milks like almond or coconut milk, and even green tea for a caffeine boost and extra antioxidants. Selecting an unsweetened liquid can help you control the overall sugar content, contributing to a healthier smoothie.

Next, we have the fruits and vegetables. Adding a diverse mix of these ingredients is essential for a nutrient-rich smoothie. Opt for antioxidant-rich fruits like blueberries, strawberries, and raspberries. These berries not only add natural sweetness but also come packed with valuable nutrients to boost your health. Don't shy away from greens either; spinach and kale are excellent choices. They provide an array of vitamins and minerals without overpowering the flavor of your smoothie.

Now, let's consider the protein source. Protein is vital for muscle repair, sustained energy, and feeling fuller for longer. Popular additions include Greek yogurt, nut butters, and protein powders. Plant-based options like hemp seeds, chia seeds, and tofu offer great alternatives for those on a vegetarian or vegan diet. Experimenting with different protein sources can help you find what works best for your taste and nutritional needs.

Then come the superfood boosters. These are the cherry on top, offering additional health benefits and unique flavors. Some excellent choices are turmeric for its anti-inflammatory properties, maca powder for improved energy and hormone balance, and spirulina for a boost of protein and essential amino acids. Each of these superfoods can elevate your smoothie from a simple snack to a nutrient powerhouse.

A perfect smoothie isn't just about what's inside the blender but also how it's prepared. Start by blending your leafy greens and liquid base first. This step ensures that the greens are finely processed, providing a smooth texture. Afterward, add fruits, followed by your protein source and superfood boosters. This layering technique helps achieve an even blend, maximizing the flavor and nutrient distribution.

Consistency is a crucial aspect of an enjoyable smoothie. If you prefer a thicker texture, incorporate ingredients like frozen fruits or a small handful of oats. Conversely, for a lighter consistency, add more liquid or use fresh fruits and vegetables. Tinkering with these elements will help you find your desired texture.

Incorporating seasonal produce can make a significant difference not only in flavor but also in nutritional value. Utilizing fresh, in-season fruits and vegetables ensures you're consuming them at their peak nutrient density. For instance, try incorporating pumpkin and apples in the fall, or berries and peaches in the summer. Seasonal variations keep your smoothie routine exciting and nutritionally beneficial all year round.

Fruit-to-vegetable ratio is another key element. A good rule of thumb is a 2:1 ratio of fruits to vegetables for a balanced taste. Too many vegetables can make the smoothie bitter, while too many fruits can spike the sugar content. Adjusting this ratio based on your preferences can result in a more enjoyable and nutritious blend.

Pay attention to sweetness levels. Natural sweeteners like honey, maple syrup, or dates can be added if extra sweetness is desired, but do so sparingly to avoid unnecessary sugar intake. Often, the natural sweetness of fruits is adequate.

Add some texture. Textural elements like chia seeds or shredded coconut can add a delightful crunch and additional nutrients. They'll also help keep you fuller for longer, making your smoothie a more substantial snack or meal replacement.

For those who require a morning energy kick, consider adding a small shot of espresso or matcha powder. These not only provide caffeine but also offer antioxidant benefits. However, keep in mind the potential for added bitterness and balance it with slight sweetness from fruits.

Don't shy away from fats. Healthy fats like avocado, flaxseed, or coconut oil can create a creamy texture and enhance the absorption of fat-soluble vitamins. These additions also provide long-lasting energy and satiety.

Finally, always taste test before serving. A quick sip can tell you if adjustments are needed. Too thick? Add more liquid. Too tart? A small banana or a splash of apple juice can make a difference. Your taste buds are your best guide in crafting the perfect smoothie blend.

Experimenting with different combinations of these components will open up a world of possibilities. Whether you prefer a tropical theme with mango and pineapple or a green goddess blend with kale, spinach, and apple, the key is to balance flavors and nutrients. The versatility of smoothies means there are endless variations to explore, ensuring that you'll never get bored and will always have a nutritious option at hand.

Chapter 17:
Medicinal Mushrooms

Medicinal mushrooms have been cherished for centuries across various cultures, prized not only for their unique flavors but also for their profound health benefits. These fungi boast an impressive array of bioactive compounds that bolster the immune system, combat oxidative stress, and support overall vitality. Reishi, often dubbed the "Mushroom of Immortality," is renowned for its immune-modulating properties, making it a staple in herbal medicine. Meanwhile, Shiitake mushrooms are celebrated for their ability to enhance immune function and offer a rich source of essential amino acids. Incorporating these fungi into your diet can be as simple as adding them to soups, stir-fries, or even brewing them into teas. Whether you're seeking to fortify your defenses against illness or simply enrich your daily meals, medicinal mushrooms provide a natural, potent pathway to better health and longevity.

Reishi: The Mushroom of Immortality

Within the realm of medicinal mushrooms, the reishi mushroom stands out for its remarkable benefits, often heralded as the "Mushroom of Immortality." This powerful fungi has been valued for centuries in various traditional medicine systems, primarily for its impressive longevity-enhancing properties. Rich in bioactive compounds, reishi aids in immune system support, reduces inflammation, and combats oxidative stress, making it an essential addition to a health-conscious lifestyle. Integration into your daily regimen can be simple; from teas and tinctures to incorporating its powdered form into smoothies or soups, reishi provides a versatile boost to overall well-being. By embracing the natural potency of this extraordinary mushroom, you're taking a significant step towards a longer, healthier life.

Integrating Reishi into Meals begins with understanding the myriad ways this fascinating superfood can elevate your everyday dishes. Known as the "Mushroom of Immortality," Reishi has been celebrated in traditional Chinese medicine for its impressive benefits, ranging from immune support to stress reduction. But how can one integrate this powerhouse into daily meals without compromising taste or culinary enjoyment? Let's explore.

One of the simplest ways to incorporate Reishi into your diet is through a finely ground powder. Reishi powder can be seamlessly added to a variety of foods and drinks. For instance, sprinkling a teaspoon into your morning smoothie isn't just an easy way to start your day with a health boost; it also camouflages the somewhat bitter taste of Reishi. Mixing it with fruits and sweeteners like banana or honey, as well as other superfoods such as spinach or chia seeds, can create a balanced and nutritious beverage that supports your health goals.

If you're a tea enthusiast, Reishi tea might become your new favorite ritual. Simply steep a piece of Reishi mushroom or a bit of Reishi powder in hot water for about 15-20 minutes. For additional flavor and benefits, consider adding a slice of ginger or a squirt of lemon. Not only will this beverage warm you up on a chilly day, but it can also fortify your immune system, making it a great option during flu season.

Beyond beverages, Reishi can play a versatile role in various meals. For instance, integrating Reishi powder into soups and stews is a brilliant way to imbue these dishes with healthful properties. Imagine a hearty mushroom and barley soup simmered with Reishi; the savory, earthy flavors meld perfectly, offering comfort and nutrition in every bite. Don't hesitate to experiment with different herbs and spices like thyme, rosemary, or bay leaves to complement the unique flavor of Reishi.

Another exciting option is integrating Reishi into your daily grain dishes. When cooking rice, quinoa, or oatmeal, try adding a small amount of Reishi powder during the cooking process. The heat helps to release the beneficial compounds from the mushroom, making your grains not only more flavorful but also more health-promoting. This method is particularly effective in savory porridge or grain bowls that can be enjoyed for breakfast, lunch, or dinner.

For those who enjoy baking, Reishi can be an unexpected yet delightful ingredient. Enrich your homemade bread, muffins, or energy bars with Reishi powder. Start with small amounts to avoid overpowering the flavor, and adjust according to your taste preference. Combining Reishi with other ingredients like dark chocolate, nuts, or dried fruits can provide a balanced and enjoyable treat that also supports your well-being.

Sauces and dressings are another clever vehicle for Reishi. Whether you're whipping up a creamy tahini dressing for a salad or a savory mushroom gravy for a holiday meal, a touch of Reishi can elevate both the nutritional profile and the flavor profile. The key is to integrate it subtly, blending it well to maintain a smooth consistency. You can also enhance these sauces with other superfoods like turmeric or garlic, creating concoctions that are as delicious as they are nourishing.

If you're into fermented foods, consider adding Reishi to your next batch of homemade kimchi or sauerkraut. The fermentation process can help mellow out some of the bitterness of the Reishi, and the combination of probiotics and adaptogenic properties can offer a comprehensive boost to your gut health and overall immunity.

Don't overlook the potential of Reishi in savory snacks and appetizers. For example, Reishi powder can be mixed with herbs and spices to create unique seasonings for roasted nuts or veggie chips. Imagine a batch of crispy kale chips seasoned with Reishi, garlic, and nutritional yeast—this not only makes for a delicious snack but also a supercharged one packed with nutrients.

Integrating Reishi doesn't have to be limited to home-cooked meals. Many stores offer Reishi-infused products like protein bars, teas, and even coffee blends. These can be convenient options for those days when time is of the essence, yet you still want to incorporate this adaptogenic mushroom into your diet.

Culinary creativity with Reishi isn't just about adding it to food for health benefits; it's also about enhancing your culinary repertoire. Reishi can be your secret ingredient in creating nutrient-dense, flavorful dishes that are both delightful and supportive of your long-term health. Remember, the key to success with Reishi—or any superfood, for that matter—is balance. Start slowly, experiment with different types of food, and find the combinations that work best for you.

To sum up, **Integrating Reishi into Meals** can be easy, delicious, and immensely beneficial for your health. From breakfast smoothies to hearty dinners and everything in between, Reishi offers a versatile way to elevate your culinary creations. So, whether you're seeking to boost your immune system, reduce stress, or simply add an extra layer of nutrition to your meals, Reishi is a powerful ally in your journey to enhanced health and longevity.

Shiitake: The Immunity Booster

Shiitake mushrooms are not just culinary delights; they provide a substantial boost to your immune system. Rich in polysaccharides, particularly the beta-glucan known as lentinan, shiitake mushrooms can enhance your body's natural defenses, helping to fend off infections and diseases. Regular consumption of these mushrooms has been scientifically linked to improved immune responses, offering protection against common colds and even more severe conditions. They're versatile in the kitchen too, easily enhancing the flavor and nutrition of various dishes, from stir-fries to soups. Integrating shiitake mushrooms into your diet is a delicious and effective way to support your overall health and longevity, making them a must-have in your superfood arsenal.

Cooking with Shiitake Mushrooms packs a punch of both flavor and health benefits. Shiitake mushrooms are known for their rich, umami taste and their impressive nutritional profile. They have been used for centuries in Asian cuisine, not only for their unique taste but also for their medicinal properties. Whether you're sautéing them as a side dish or adding them to a hearty stew, shiitake mushrooms can elevate any meal while boosting your health.

When it comes to cooking with shiitake mushrooms, the possibilities are virtually endless. Start with the basics: fresh and dried shiitake mushrooms. Fresh shiitakes have a more delicate texture and flavor, while dried shiitakes are often more concentrated in taste. Rehydrating dried shiitakes is simple—just soak them in warm water for about 20 minutes. Not only does this make them tender, but the soaking liquid can be used as a flavorful broth for soups and sauces.

One of the easiest ways to enjoy shiitake mushrooms is by sautéing them. Heat some olive oil in a pan, add sliced shiitakes, and cook until they are golden brown. Season with garlic, salt, and pepper to taste. Adding a splash of soy sauce or tamari can elevate their umami profile even further. Serve them as a topping for salads, pizzas, or even burgers. The rich texture and flavor can also complement a variety of proteins, including tofu, chicken, and beef.

Shiitake mushrooms shine in soups and stews. Their meaty texture allows them to hold up well during long cooking times, infusing the dishes with their earthy flavor. Try adding them to miso soup, where they pair beautifully with the soy-based broth and tofu. For a heartier option, consider a shiitake mushroom and barley soup. Sauté onions, carrots, and celery, then add shiitake mushrooms, vegetable broth, barley, and your choice of herbs and spices. Simmer until the barley is tender and the mushrooms have imparted their rich flavor into the soup.

For those looking to experiment, shiitake mushrooms can also be used in more complex dishes like risottos and pastas. Their deep, savory notes can enhance the flavors of creamy risottos or simple pasta dishes. Cook them with onions and garlic, then mix them into a creamy risotto or Alfredo sauce. The mushrooms' natural umami will make the dish deeply satisfying without the need for heavy creams or excessive cheese.

Not to be overlooked, shiitake mushrooms are also excellent in stir-fries. Their quick cooking time makes them perfect for this high-heat method. Combine them with other nutrient-dense vegetables like bell peppers, broccoli, and snap peas. Add a bit of ginger and garlic for an extra punch of flavor, and finish with a splash of soy sauce or hoisin sauce. Serve over steamed brown rice or quinoa for a complete, nutritious meal.

Shiitake mushrooms can also be incorporated into grain bowls and salads for a quick and nutritious meal. For a grain bowl, layer cooked quinoa or brown rice with roasted vegetables, avocado slices, and sautéed shiitake mushrooms. Drizzle with a tahini or miso-based dressing for added flavor. For salads, consider using raw shiitake mushrooms thinly sliced or marinated in a mixture of olive oil, lemon juice, and herbs. Their unique texture and taste can turn a simple salad into a gourmet experience.

In addition to their culinary versatility, shiitake mushrooms offer a host of health benefits. They are rich in B vitamins, including B2, B5, and B6, which are essential for energy production and overall metabolic function. They are also a good source of copper, selenium, and zinc, minerals that contribute to a healthy immune system. The compounds found in shiitake mushrooms, such as lentinan and eritadenine, have been studied for their potential anti-cancer and cholesterol-lowering properties.

For a more exotic twist, try making shiitake mushroom sushi rolls. Use the rehydrated mushrooms as a filling along with cucumber, avocado, and a smear of wasabi. The mushrooms' meaty texture pairs well with the fresh, crisp vegetables, making for a satisfying and nutritious sushi experience.

Baking enthusiasts can also find ways to incorporate shiitake mushrooms into their recipes. Consider making a savory shiitake mushroom and herb bread. The mushrooms add moisture and a deep, savory flavor to the bread, making it a perfect accompaniment to soups and stews. Simply sauté the mushrooms with some garlic and herbs, then mix them into your bread dough before baking.

For breakfast, shiitake mushrooms can be a game-changer. Add sautéed shiitakes to your morning omelet or scramble for a protein-packed start to your day. Pair them with spinach, tomatoes, and a sprinkle of feta cheese for extra flavor. They also work well in breakfast bowls, mixed with quinoa, black beans, avocado, and a poached egg.

Another delicious way to use shiitake mushrooms is by making a mushroom pâté. Blend sautéed shiitakes with garlic, thyme, and olive oil until smooth. This can be served on toast or crackers as an appetizer or snack. The pâté's rich flavor and creamy texture make it a delightful addition to any meal.

To make sure you're getting the most out of your shiitake mushrooms, always opt for organic varieties when possible. Many commercial mushrooms can be treated with chemicals, so organic options are typically better for both your health and the environment.

While freshly prepared dishes are fantastic, don't underestimate the utility of shiitake mushrooms in meal prep. Cook a big batch of sautéed shiitakes at the beginning of the week and add them to various meals throughout. They can be kept in the refrigerator for up to five days and swiftly integrated into quick lunches and dinners, such as wraps, grain bowls, and even as a topping for homemade pizzas.

So, as you embark on your journey to a healthier lifestyle, don't forget to keep shiitake mushrooms in your culinary arsenal. With their versatility, rich flavor, and impressive health benefits, they are an indispensable addition to any diet aimed at enhancing longevity and well-being. Whether you're a seasoned chef or a kitchen newbie, there's always a delicious, nutritious way to include shiitake mushrooms in your meals.

Chapter 18:
Exotic Superfoods

In this chapter, we uncover the hidden gems of the superfood world, presenting you with vibrant and nutrient-rich choices that hail from the far corners of the globe. From the nutrient-dense acai berries of the Amazon rainforest to the antioxidant-loaded goji berries cherished in traditional Chinese medicine, these exotic superfoods are not only delicious but also pack a powerful punch for your health. Discover how these unique offerings can elevate your diet, providing benefits ranging from enhanced immunity to increased energy levels. Integrating these superfoods into your daily routine can be as simple as sprinkling them on your morning oatmeal or blending them into your smoothies. Each of these ingredients has a story, a heritage of health that has been celebrated for centuries, and now, they can easily become a part of your modern, health-conscious lifestyle.

Acai: The Amazonian Super Berry

Hailing from the lush rainforests of the Amazon, acai berries have earned their place in the superfood hall of fame for good reason. These small, dark purple fruits are packed with an impressive blend of antioxidants, fiber, and heart-healthy fats. More than just a trendy smoothie ingredient, acai berries have been a dietary staple for indigenous Amazonian tribes for centuries, providing them with a sustained source of energy, vitality, and immune support. The high concentration of anthocyanins in acai berries helps combat oxidative stress and inflammation, making them a potent ally in the fight against chronic diseases. When looking to elevate your health regimen, consider integrating acai berries into your diet to harness their myriad of benefits and bring a taste of the Amazon into your daily nutrition.

Incorporating Acai into Breakfast can be both an exciting and rewarding endeavor. Acai, the Amazonian super berry, has gained a considerable amount of popularity in recent years—and for good reason. Packed with antioxidants, fiber, and heart-healthy fats, it's a powerful food that can be seamlessly integrated into your morning routine, giving you the perfect boost to start your day on a healthy note.

One of the simplest ways to enjoy acai for breakfast is by making an acai bowl. These vibrant bowls combine frozen acai puree with a variety of fruits, granola, and seeds. Start by blending frozen acai packets with a bit of almond milk or coconut water to get a thick, sorbet-like consistency. You can also toss in frozen bananas or berries for added flavor and texture. Pour the mixture into a bowl and top it off with your favorite fruits like sliced bananas, strawberries, blueberries, chia seeds, and a drizzle of honey or agave syrup.

If you prefer something more portable, acai smoothies could be your go-to. Blend acai pulp with ingredients like spinach, kale, banana, and almond milk. Adding a scoop of protein powder or a tablespoon of nut butter can make it more filling and provide extra nutrients. This not only makes for a delicious breakfast but also a great post-workout snack.

For those who like a bit more variety, try incorporating acai into your breakfast parfaits. Layer acai puree with Greek yogurt, mixed berries, and granola in a glass or jar. This layered dessert-like breakfast is not only visually appealing but also packs a nutrient punch, giving you essential vitamins and minerals to kickstart your day.

You don't have to eat acai bowls or smoothies every day to make the most of this superfood. Another option is to sprinkle acai powder over your morning oatmeal. This is a particularly good choice in colder months when warm breakfasts are more appealing. Simply prepare your oatmeal as usual, then mix in a teaspoon of acai powder, and top with fresh fruit and nuts for added texture and nutrients.

For those who enjoy baking, consider adding acai to your breakfast muffins or pancakes. Acai powder can be mixed into the batter, giving your baked goods a nutritional boost along with a hint of berry flavor. Use whole grain flour, almond flour, or oats as the base to create a truly wholesome breakfast treat.

Sometimes, innovating with acai can lead to new breakfast staples. For instance, acai chia pudding can be a delightful way to switch things up. Mix chia seeds, almond milk, and acai powder, then let it sit overnight in the refrigerator. By morning, you'll have a delicious, pudding-like consistency that's ready to be topped with fruits, nuts, or a spoonful of nut butter.

Not only does acai elevate the nutritional profile of these breakfasts, but it also adds a burst of color and flavor that's hard to resist. The berry boasts an impressive ORAC (Oxygen Radical Absorbance Capacity) value, making it one of the top antioxidant-rich foods available. A diet rich in antioxidants can help combat free radicals, which are harmful molecules that can contribute to cellular damage and aging.

Another practical tip is to prepare and store acai mixes ahead of time. For instance, pre-blend your smoothie mixes and freeze them in individual portions. In the morning, all you need to do is blend them with your choice of liquid, and you have a nutritious breakfast ready in minutes. This can be particularly useful for busy mornings when time is of the essence.

Moreover, incorporating acai into your breakfast doesn't have to stop at traditional dishes. Be creative and experiment with different recipes. For example, try acai breakfast bars made with a mix of oats, nuts, seeds, and acai powder. These can be baked and stored, offering a grab-and-go option that's both healthy and convenient.

It's also important to balance the acai with other nutrient-dense foods to ensure a well-rounded meal. Combining it with protein sources like Greek yogurt, nut butter, or even eggs can help sustain energy levels throughout the morning. Adding healthy fats from sources like avocado or nuts will also enhance the absorption of fat-soluble vitamins in your breakfast.

Incorporating acai into breakfast can revolutionize your morning routine, enhancing both flavor and nutritional intake. Whether you choose to enjoy it in a bowl, smoothie, parfait, or any other creative dish, acai's versatility ensures you won't tire of it anytime soon. Start experimenting today and experience the myriad benefits this Amazonian berry has to offer.

Goji Berries: The Red Diamond

Highly prized in traditional Chinese medicine, goji berries offer a unique blend of nutrients that make them a must-add to your superfood arsenal. These small but mighty red berries are rich in antioxidants, particularly zeaxanthin, which is known to protect eye health. Additionally, they are a great source of essential amino acids and polysaccharides, which support immune function and overall vitality. Incorporating goji berries into your daily routine can be as simple as adding them to your morning smoothie, sprinkling them over a salad, or even snacking on a handful. With their slightly sweet and tangy flavor, goji berries not only enhance your meals but also provide a potent boost of nutrients that your body will thank you for.

Goji Berry Snack Ideas Goji berries, often called "red diamonds," are one of the most potent superfoods you can incorporate into your diet. These small, bright red berries are packed with nutrients and antioxidants, making them an excellent choice for anyone looking to boost their health and longevity. But how do you make the most out of these nutrient-rich gems? Let's explore some delicious and creative snack ideas that make goji berries a versatile addition to your daily routine.

First up, a simple and delightful way to enjoy goji berries is by adding them to trail mix. Trail mix is a timeless snack, perfect for on-the-go munching or a quick post-workout boost. Combine goji berries with a mix of raw almonds, cashews, pumpkin seeds, and a sprinkle of dark chocolate chips. The natural sweetness of the goji berries pairs perfectly with the crunch of the nuts and seeds, while the dark chocolate provides a hint of indulgence. This mix not only tastes great but also provides a balanced blend of protein, healthy fats, and antioxidants.

For those who love yogurt, goji berries make a fantastic topping. Stir a handful of these berries into your favorite Greek yogurt for a nutrient-packed breakfast or a satisfying snack. You can enhance the flavor by adding a dash of honey, some chia seeds, and a few slices of fresh fruit like strawberries or bananas. Not only does this combination taste divine, but it also offers a powerhouse of nutrients, including protein, fiber, and vitamins.

If you're fond of smoothies, goji berries can easily be integrated into your blends. A fruity goji berry smoothie is simple to make: blend a handful of goji berries with a banana, a cup of frozen berries, a handful of spinach, and some almond milk. For an added protein boost, throw in a scoop of your favorite protein powder. This smoothie is a refreshing and vibrant way to start your day, providing you with essential nutrients and energy to power through your morning.

Another innovative way to enjoy goji berries is by incorporating them into homemade energy bars. These bars are incredibly easy to make and are a perfect portable snack. In a food processor, blend dates, goji berries, oats, almonds, and a bit of coconut oil until the mixture comes together. Press the mixture into a baking dish and refrigerate until firm. Once set, cut into bars or squares. These bars provide a chewy, satisfying texture and are packed with nutrients to keep you fueled throughout the day.

For a savory twist, consider making goji berry and quinoa salad. Cooked quinoa acts as a perfect base for various ingredients, and goji berries add a touch of sweetness, balancing the flavors beautifully. Combine cooked quinoa with chopped kale, diced avocado, cherry tomatoes, and a handful of goji berries. Toss the salad with a light lemon vinaigrette made from lemon juice, olive oil, and a pinch of salt. This salad is not only colorful but also brimming with essential nutrients, fiber, and healthy fats.

Boots of morning muffins with a nutritional punch by adding some goji berries to your batter. These berries can be used similarly to raisins or dried cranberries in baking. Mix them into a whole grain muffin batter along with other ingredients like oats, nuts, and spices such as cinnamon or nutmeg. Bake until golden brown, and you'll have delicious, nutritious muffins perfect for breakfast or a midday snack.

A delightful dessert option is goji berry chia pudding. Chia pudding is known for its creamy texture and high nutrient content, and goji berries make it even better. To prepare this treat, soak chia seeds in almond milk or coconut milk overnight, stirring occasionally to prevent clumping. In the morning, mix in a handful of rehydrated goji berries, a drizzle of honey or maple syrup, and a splash of vanilla extract. This pudding can be enjoyed as a rich breakfast or a healthy dessert.

Goji berries also make an excellent addition to homemade granola. Mix oats with a variety of nuts and seeds, then coat the mixture with a blend of honey, coconut oil, and a touch of vanilla extract. Bake until golden and crispy, then stir in a generous amount of goji berries. This granola can be enjoyed with yogurt, milk, or even on its own as a crunchy snack.

Fancy a goji berry tea? You can easily make a warm, soothing drink by steeping a handful of goji berries in hot water for about 10-15 minutes. Add a slice of lemon, a piece of fresh ginger, and a touch of honey for added flavor. This tea is not only refreshing but also provides a mild, sweet flavor and a significant antioxidant boost.

Incorporating goji berries into savory dishes can be quite intriguing. For instance, you can add them to a stir-fry. Sauté your favorite vegetables and either tofu or chicken in a bit of olive oil, then toss in a handful of goji berries towards the end of cooking. The goji berries will rehydrate, adding a burst of sweetness that complements the savory flavors of the stir-fry.

Another savory approach is to mix goji berries into a grain bowl. Combine cooked grains like farro or brown rice with roasted vegetables, chickpeas, and a handful of goji berries. Drizzle with a tahini dressing or your favorite vinaigrette. This dish merges different textures and flavors, providing a wholesome and satisfying meal.

For those who enjoy experimenting in the kitchen, goji berry-infused sauces can be a real marvel. Blend goji berries with a bit of water, lemon juice, garlic, and olive oil to create a tangy, antioxidant-rich sauce. This can be drizzled over salads, grilled meats, or roasted vegetables for an extra layer of flavor and nutrition.

Lastly, don't forget about baking! Incorporate goji berries into cakes, cookies, and bread for a nutrient-dense twist on your favorite recipes. Next time you're baking banana bread, add in a handful of goji berries alongside the nuts and chocolate chips for a deliciously unique flavor.

Trail mix with goji berries

Yogurt topped with goji berries, chia seeds, and fresh fruit

Fruit smoothies with goji berries

Homemade energy bars featuring goji berries

Quinoa salad with goji berries and avocado

Whole grain muffins with goji berries

Goji berry chia pudding

Homemade granola with goji berries

Goji berry tea

Savory stir-fry with goji berries

Grain bowls with goji berries

Goji berry-infused sauces

Baked goods with goji berries

These diverse and delicious snack ideas demonstrate that there are countless ways

Chapter 19:
Healthy Desserts

Indulging your sweet tooth doesn't have to derail your health goals, and "Healthy Desserts" proves just that. By focusing on nutrient-dense superfoods, you can create decadent treats that also provide essential vitamins, minerals, and antioxidants. Imagine biting into a rich, dark chocolate truffle packed with flavonoids or savoring a bowl of fresh berries topped with creamy Greek yogurt, each spoonful delivering probiotics and fiber. These desserts not only satisfy your cravings but also give your body a boost, maintaining energy levels and supporting overall well-being. With a few creative twists and some thoughtful ingredient choices, you can enjoy guilt-free desserts that contribute to your longevity and health in delightful ways.

Dark Chocolate: The Guilt-Free Treat

When it comes to indulgent snacks that also harbor significant health benefits, dark chocolate stands as an unrivaled champion. Unlike its milk chocolate counterpart, dark chocolate is rich in antioxidants, particularly flavonoids, which have been shown to enhance blood flow, reduce blood pressure, and improve overall heart health. What's more, dark chocolate can elevate your mood by stimulating the brain's production of endorphins and serotonin. Incorporating a modest portion of high-quality dark chocolate—ideally with a cocoa content of 70% or higher—into your diet can provide not just a satisfying treat, but also a valuable boost to your health and longevity. So go ahead, enjoy a piece of dark chocolate without the guilt, knowing you're doing your body a favor.

Dark Chocolate Dessert Recipes combine the richness of dark chocolate with the health benefits it notoriously carries. Dark chocolate, especially varieties with high cocoa content, is loaded with antioxidants and has been linked to numerous health benefits, including heart health and improved brain function. This section will guide you through a selection of delectable, nutrient-dense dessert recipes, ensuring you can savor your sweet tooth without compromising your health goals.

Incorporating dark chocolate into your dessert repertoire can be as simple or as sophisticated as you like. For those who enjoy the pure essence of chocolate, a classic dark chocolate bark might be the perfect choice. To make it, all you need is some high-quality dark chocolate (preferably 70% cocoa or higher), and your choice of mix-ins such as nuts, seeds, and dried fruit. Melt the chocolate, pour it onto a parchment-lined baking sheet, sprinkle your chosen toppings, and let it set in the refrigerator. This easy and customizable treat can also make a great gift!

If you're looking for something a bit more indulgent, why not try a dark chocolate avocado mousse? This dessert leverages the creamy texture of ripe avocados to create a rich and smooth mousse that's also packed with healthy fats. Simply blend ripe avocados with melted dark chocolate, a splash of almond milk, and a touch of vanilla extract until smooth. Sweeten it with a bit of honey or maple syrup to taste. Not only does this mousse deliver on creaminess, but it also supplies a good dose of vitamins and minerals from the avocados.

Certainly, another crowd-pleaser that's both nutritious and delicious is the dark chocolate chia pudding. Chia seeds are known for their omega-3 fatty acids, fiber, and protein, making them an ideal superfood. To prepare this pudding, mix chia seeds with almond milk, cocoa powder, and a natural sweetener of your choice. Stir well and let the mixture sit in the fridge overnight. The chia seeds will absorb the liquid and form a pudding-like consistency. Top it off with fresh berries or a sprinkle of crushed nuts for added texture and flavor.

For a dessert that feels a little more traditional yet still health-conscious, consider baking a dark chocolate olive oil cake. Olive oil not only adds moisture but also imparts a subtle and rich flavor that's complemented by dark chocolate. Combine flour, cocoa powder, baking soda, and a pinch of salt in a bowl. In another bowl, whisk together olive oil, a couple of eggs, coconut sugar, and vanilla extract. Mix the wet and dry ingredients together and fold in chopped dark chocolate chunks before pouring the batter into a cake tin. Bake until a toothpick inserted into the center comes out clean. The result is a moist, flavorful cake that's perfect for any occasion.

Lastly, for those who need a quick and easy treat, dark chocolate-covered strawberries are hard to beat. Simply melt some dark chocolate and dip fresh, organic strawberries into it. Lay them out on a parchment-lined tray and let them harden in the fridge. These make for an antioxidant-packed dessert that's both visually stunning and incredibly tasty.

While these recipes are delicious and healthy, it's essential to note that the quality of the dark chocolate you use plays a crucial role. Always opt for chocolate that has at least 70% cocoa content and check for minimal added sugars and no artificial additives. Organic and fair-trade options are preferable as they often ensure higher quality ingredients and better farming practices.

Not only do these dark chocolate desserts provide a healthier option to satisfy sweet cravings, but they also allow you to enjoy the multifaceted benefits of dark chocolate. From its heart-friendly flavonoids to its potential in improving cognitive function, dark chocolate, when consumed mindfully, can be a valuable addition to your diet. So, next time you're in the mood for dessert, consider these recipes as guilt-free and health-boosting options.

Whether you are entertaining guests or simply treating yourself, these dark chocolate dessert recipes can be seamlessly integrated into your daily life. They demonstrate that healthy eating doesn't have to sacrifice flavor or enjoyment. By choosing nutrient-dense ingredients, you create desserts that nourish your body while indulging your palate. Enjoy the best of both worlds with these thoughtfully crafted recipes and make superfoods a delightful part of your culinary journey.

As you experiment with these recipes, don't hesitate to get creative. Add your favorite superfoods like a sprinkle of hemp seeds, a dusting of maca powder, or a hint of turmeric to enhance both the flavor and nutritional profile of your desserts. The flexibility of dark chocolate as an ingredient means it pairs beautifully with a wide variety of other superfoods, allowing for endless variations and new culinary discoveries.

In conclusion, **Dark Chocolate Dessert Recipes** offer a luscious pathway to delicious and health-boosting indulgence. By selecting quality ingredients and experimenting with nutrient-dense additions, you can make desserts that are not only a treat to your taste buds but also a boon to your health. Revel in these recipes and enjoy the profound satisfaction of desserts that are both delightful and nourishing.

Berries with Greek Yogurt: Simple and Nutritious

For a dessert that's as delicious as it is beneficial, look no further than a bowl of berries with Greek yogurt. This simple combination effortlessly melds the antioxidant-rich power of berries with the protein-packed goodness of Greek yogurt. Rich in vitamins, minerals, and gut-friendly probiotics, Greek yogurt serves as an excellent base, enhancing the natural sweetness and tartness of the berries. Whether you choose blueberries, strawberries, or raspberries, you'll create a vibrant, nutrient-dense treat that's perfect for any time of day. Best of all, it's quick to prepare and easily customizable—drizzle a bit of honey or sprinkle some chia seeds for added texture and flavor. This wholesome pairing not only satisfies your sweet tooth but also fuels your body with essential nutrients, making it an ideal choice for anyone aiming to elevate their health and longevity through superfoods.

Creative Dessert Ideas In the quest to incorporate superfoods into every meal, it's easy to believe desserts might pose a challenge. However, with a bit of creativity, they become an exciting venue for nutrient-dense delights. After all, who says indulgence can't also be beneficial? This section will guide you through innovative and delightful ways to transform everyday desserts into superfood-rich creations that not only satisfy your sweet tooth but also contribute to your health and longevity.

Think about the classic combination of berries and Greek yogurt. Adding a drizzle of honey and a sprinkling of chia seeds not only boosts the nutrient profile but also enhances the texture and flavor. Start with fresh, antioxidant-packed berries like blueberries, strawberries, and raspberries. These berries are low in calories yet high in vitamins, minerals, and fiber. Pair them with Greek yogurt, which is rich in protein and probiotics, and you've got a simple but powerful dessert.

For a slight spin on this, consider making a layered parfait. Begin with a base of Greek yogurt, add a layer of mixed berries, then sprinkle in some raw walnuts or almonds for added crunch and healthy fats. Alternate these layers until you reach the top of your serving dish, finishing off with a dollop of yogurt and a garnish of fresh mint. This parfait not only looks stunning but is a nutrient powerhouse thanks to the combination of protein, healthy fats, fiber, and antioxidants.

If you're a fan of chocolate, there are numerous ways to enjoy this treat while enhancing its health benefits. Dark chocolate, particularly those varieties with 70% cacao content or higher, is rich in antioxidants called flavonoids. These compounds are known to help lower blood pressure and improve vascular function. One creative dessert idea is dark chocolate avocado mousse. The creaminess of ripe avocados blends seamlessly with the rich flavor of dark chocolate, providing a dessert that's both decadent and nutritious.

To make this mousse, blend ripe avocados with melted dark chocolate, a splash of almond milk, and a bit of vanilla extract. Sweeten it to taste with a natural sweetener like maple syrup or honey. This mousse not only benefits from the antioxidants in the dark chocolate but also the healthy monounsaturated fats from the avocado, which are great for heart health!

Another creamy delight can be created with cashew cream, a versatile base for many desserts. Soak cashews in water until they are soft, then blend them with a touch of vanilla extract, lemon juice, and a natural sweetener. This can be used as a topping for fresh fruit or as a filling for no-bake tarts. Consider pairing it with a date and nut crust for a raw, nutrient-rich treat. Dates are packed with natural sugars, fiber, and various vitamins and minerals, while nuts provide protein and healthy fats.

Speaking of no-bake desserts, superfood energy balls are a popular option that packs a lot of nutrition into a small bite. These energy balls can be made by blending oats, nut butter, honey, and your choice of superfood additions. Chia seeds, flaxseeds, and goji berries all make excellent choices. Roll the mixture into balls and refrigerate until firm. These bite-sized treats are perfect for a quick snack or a post-dinner delight.

For fruit lovers, transforming a simple fruit salad into a superfood-rich dessert is effortless. Combine a variety of your favorite fruits –

think mangoes, kiwis, blueberries, and pomegranates. Add a handful of chopped nuts and seeds like almonds, walnuts, or pumpkin seeds for crunch and additional nutrients. Drizzle a light dressing made from fresh orange juice and a bit of honey over the top. This colorful dish is not only visually appealing but also rich in vitamins, minerals, and healthy fats.

If you're inclined to bake, muffins and breads can easily incorporate superfoods. For example, blueberry chia muffins blend the antioxidant power of blueberries with the omega-3 richness of chia seeds. Use whole grain flour for additional fiber and nutrients. Alternatively, sweet potato brownies make a decadent dessert loaded with beta-carotene, vitamins, and minerals. Sweet potatoes add natural sweetness, meaning you can reduce the amount of added sugar in your recipe.

Another baked delight is almond flour cookies. Almond flour is gluten-free and high in protein and healthy fats. Mix almond flour with dark chocolate chips, a bit of coconut oil, and a natural sweetener to create cookies that are both nutritious and satisfying. For an additional nutrient boost, consider adding a tablespoon of maca powder, which is known for its energy-boosting properties.

When crunched for time, frozen desserts offer a quick and healthy alternative. One simple idea is to make your own superfood ice pops. Blend ingredients like Greek yogurt, mixed berries, some spinach (the flavor blends well and goes unnoticed), and a bit of honey. Pour the mixture into ice pop molds and freeze. These refreshing treats are perfect for hot days and offer numerous health benefits in a convenient form.

Smoothie bowls are another frozen treat that's customizable and loaded with superfoods. Blend a combination of frozen fruits such as acai berries, bananas, and strawberries with a bit of almond milk until thick and creamy. Pour the mixture into a bowl and top with your favorite nutritious extras. Chia seeds, sliced fruits, granola, coconut flakes, and even a drizzle of nut butter make excellent toppings. This dessert is both satisfying and bursting with vitamins, minerals, and antioxidants.

For a summer favorite, consider grilling fruits like peaches or pineapples. Grilling caramelizes the natural sugars, enhancing their sweetness. Pair with a scoop of Greek yogurt and a sprinkle of nuts for a well-rounded dessert. Pineapples are packed with vitamin C, while peaches provide a good source of vitamins A and E, making this dish a nutritional triumph.

Lastly, let's not forget the traditional treat of homemade granola. It's extremely versatile and can be used as a topping for yogurt, smoothie bowls, or enjoyed on its own. To make superfood granola, combine oats with a mix of nuts and seeds - almonds, chia seeds, and flaxseeds are all stellar choices. Sweeten with a bit of honey or maple syrup, and add dried fruits like blueberries or cranberries. Bake until golden and crunchy. Granola is excellent for a breakfast parfait or an anytime snack, and it keeps well stored in an airtight container.

Incorporating superfoods into your desserts doesn't mean compromising on taste or satisfaction. By experimenting with combinations and using nutrient-rich ingredients, you can create a variety of desserts that are both delicious and beneficial for your health. As you explore these creative ideas, you'll find that the boundary between indulgence and nutrition becomes delightfully blurred.

Chapter 20:
Practical Tips for Superfoods

Incorporating superfoods into your daily routine can transform your health, but knowing where to start can be daunting. To make it simpler, start by shopping smart—opt for local and seasonal produce where possible, and always check for vibrant colors and firm textures to ensure maximum freshness. Planning your meals ahead not only saves time but also ensures a balanced diet rich in diverse superfoods. Prepare a weekly meal plan that includes a variety of fruits, vegetables, grains, and legumes to cover all nutritional bases. Focus on simple recipes that emphasize the natural flavors of these nutrient-dense foods. When shopping, consider bulk buying of versatile staples like quinoa and lentils, which can serve as the foundation for many meals. Lastly, always keep some easy-to-prepare superfoods like leafy greens and berries on hand for quick, nutritious snacks that can seamlessly fit into any busy lifestyle.

Shopping Smart for Superfoods

When it comes to shopping smart for superfoods, the key is to focus on freshness, seasonality, and quality. Start by frequenting local farmers' markets where you can find nutrient-rich produce that's often grown organically, ensuring maximum health benefits. Always look for bright colors and firm textures, which usually indicate the highest levels of nutrients. Don't hesitate to ask vendors about their farming practices or the origin of their products; understanding where your food comes from can help you make more informed choices. Learning how to read labels effectively can also make a world of difference; prioritize products with minimal additives and check for any certifications that indicate sustainable practices. Shopping with a list tailored to your health goals can keep you focused and more likely to make nutritious choices. Additionally, buying in bulk for non-perishables like quinoa or almonds can save money while ensuring you always have superfoods on hand. Remember, investing a bit of time and effort into your grocery shopping can yield substantial health dividends.

Tips for Selecting Fresh Produce are essential for anyone looking to enrich their diet with nutrient-dense superfoods. The key to maximizing the health benefits of fruits and vegetables lies in choosing the freshest options available. Fresh produce not only tastes better but also boasts higher nutritional content. Here's how to get started in making the best selections at the grocery store, farmer's market, or even your own backyard garden.

First, it's crucial to understand the importance of seasonality. Produce that is in season is usually fresher, cheaper, and more nutritious. Seasonal fruits and vegetables are typically harvested at their peak ripeness and don't need to travel long distances, thus retaining more nutrients. For example, strawberries in the summer are a whole different experience compared to the off-season varieties. Always aim to buy what's in season, and your body will thank you.

Another vital tip is to know the tell-tale signs of freshness for various types of produce. Look for fruits and vegetables with vibrant, rich colors. Dull or faded hues can indicate that the item is past its prime. A bright green spinach leaf or a deep orange carrot suggests the presence of various phytochemicals and vitamins. In contrast, pale or yellowing leaves may signify nutrient loss.

Texture is also a good indicator of freshness. Firmness in fruits like apples, peaches, and pears suggests that they are fresh. A gently firm squeeze should have a bit of give, but if it's too soft and mushy, it's likely overripe. On the flip side, if it's rock-hard, it might not have ripened properly. For leafy greens like kale and spinach, the leaves should be crisp and free from wilting or browning edges.

Your sense of smell can be a useful tool when selecting fresh produce. Many fruits emit a sweet, fragrant aroma when they are at peak ripeness. For example, a ripe mango or melon will have a noticeable, pleasant smell. If fruit lacks any scent, it may lack flavor as well.

Lastly, consider the source of your produce. Local and organic options are generally fresher because they haven't traveled far from the farm to your table. When buying from a farmer's market, don't hesitate to ask the vendors about their farming practices and the freshness of their produce. Many farmers are happy to share information about when and how their crops were harvested.

Buying organic is another important factor. Organic produce is cultivated without synthetic pesticides or fertilizers, making it a healthier choice for your body and the environment. While organic options might be more expensive, some items, such as leafy greens, berries, and apples, are particularly worth buying organic due to their high pesticide residue levels when conventionally grown. Consider using resources like the Environmental Working Group's Dirty Dozen and Clean Fifteen lists to prioritize which fruits and vegetables to buy organic.

Be mindful of storage and handling to maintain the freshness of your produce after purchase. Different types of fruits and vegetables have varying storage requirements. For example, tomatoes prefer room temperature storage away from direct sunlight, while leafy greens should be kept in the refrigerator to stay crisp and fresh. Using breathable produce bags or containers can also extend the life of your fresh items.

While shopping, always examine produce closely at multiple points along your grocery journey. This means from the moment you pick it up in-store to when you're washing it at home. Inspect for any signs of mold, bruises, or blemishes. These flaws can lead to quicker spoilage and diminished nutritional value.

If you find yourself with an abundance of fresh produce that you can't consume right away, consider freezing it for later use. Flash-freezing fruits like berries and vegetables like broccoli retains much of the nutritional content and extends their shelf life. Simply wash, dry thoroughly, and freeze in a single layer before transferring them to airtight containers or freezer bags.

Don't overlook the benefits of growing your own produce if you have space and time. Homegrown fruits and vegetables can be harvested at peak ripeness, ensuring they are as fresh and nutrient-packed as possible. Even a small herb garden can provide fresh flavors and extra nutrients to your meals.

When selecting fresh produce, your senses of sight, touch, and smell will guide you well. Prioritizing organic and seasonal items, understanding storage needs, and considering local sources will further enhance the freshness and nutritional value of your choices. By doing so, you'll be well on your way to harnessing the full power of superfoods for your health and longevity.

Meal Planning with Superfoods

Integrating superfoods into your daily meal plan doesn't have to be challenging or time-consuming. Start by selecting a variety of superfoods that align with your dietary preferences and health goals. Opt for a colorful mix of antioxidant-rich fruits, leafy greens, and whole grains to create balanced, nutrient-dense meals that provide sustained energy and support overall well-being. For instance, you can kick off the day with a quinoa breakfast bowl topped with fresh berries and chia seeds, and enjoy a kale and spinach salad for lunch, garnished with almonds and a drizzle of olive oil. Dinner could be a hearty lentil soup accompanied by a side of roasted sweet potatoes. The key is to keep your meals diverse and exciting, experimenting with different superfoods and recipes to discover what works best for you. By planning your meals in advance and incorporating superfoods seamlessly, you'll find it easier to maintain a healthy and vibrant lifestyle.

Creating Balanced Meal Plans is essential for anyone aiming to incorporate nutrient-dense superfoods into their daily diets. The foundation of a balanced meal plan lies in ensuring that every meal provides a variety of nutrients to support overall health and longevity. By integrating superfoods, one can amplify the nutritional content of meals without compromising on taste or satisfaction.

A balanced meal plan includes an appropriate mix of macronutrients: proteins, carbohydrates, and fats, alongside essential vitamins and minerals. Each meal should ideally contain a serving of protein, whole grains or complex carbohydrates, and healthy fats. To achieve this, it's crucial to include a diverse range of superfoods. For instance, you could pair quinoa, a complete protein, with a leafy green salad topped with a handful of antioxidant-rich berries and a drizzle of olive oil. This not only covers the macronutrients but also supplies a spectrum of micronutrients.

Superfoods are not a separate food group but can be integrated into every meal. For breakfast, consider starting with a smoothie made from a mix of fruits like blueberries and chia seeds. These are not just nutrient-dense but also provide a good balance of fiber, antioxidants, and omega-3 fatty acids. Adding spinach to your smoothie is an excellent way to introduce leafy greens early in your day.

For lunch, think about a bowl that combines various superfoods. A quinoa and kale salad topped with pomegranate seeds, almonds, and a squeeze of lemon juice can be both filling and extremely nourishing. This combination ensures a good mix of protein, fiber, healthy fats, and a range of vitamins and minerals that support overall health. The key is variety; each ingredient brings its unique set of nutrients.

Dinner should be an opportunity to incorporate more superfoods. A dish featuring salmon, which is rich in omega-3 fatty acids, paired with a side of steamed broccoli and a serving of sweet potatoes, offers a wealth of health benefits. Each component of this meal works together to provide essential nutrients while keeping the palate engaged with different tastes and textures.

Transitioning from individual meals, let's look into the weekly perspective. Planning meals at the beginning of the week can ensure a balanced intake of nutrients without the stress of daily decision-making. A well-planned week can rotate different superfoods to keep the diet exciting and nutritionally rich.

Begin with a template that includes diverse superfoods across all meals. Aim for something like this: Breakfasts could alternate between smoothies, chia seed puddings, and oatmeal topped with fruits like raspberries and nuts. Lunches might rotate between grain bowls, hearty salads, or wraps filled with legumes like lentils or chickpeas, and a variety of vegetables. Dinners can feature different protein sources such as salmon, legumes, or tofu, paired with whole grains and a mix of vegetables, either raw or cooked.

Don't forget about snacks. They are vital in maintaining energy levels throughout the day and can be a strategic way to include more superfoods. Snack ideas can include a handful of almonds, a piece of fruit, or a small dish of yogurt topped with goji berries. Homemade protein balls made with seeds and nuts are another great option.

Balancing flavors and textures also plays a critical role in meal satisfaction. Superfoods often bring intense flavors and unique textures. Balancing bitter kale with sweet berries, or the crunch of almonds with the creaminess of avocados, can create a more enjoyable and satisfying eating experience.

While focusing on individual superfoods is important, the notion of synergy should not be overlooked. Certain combinations of foods can enhance nutrient absorption. For example, pairing vitamin C-rich foods like strawberries or lemons with iron-rich foods like spinach can significantly boost iron absorption. Similarly, fat-soluble vitamins found in vegetables can be better absorbed when consumed with a source of healthy fat, such as olive oil or avocado.

Creating balanced meal plans also means being mindful of portion sizes and overall dietary patterns. Eating a variety of superfoods in appropriate quantities ensures that the body gets all necessary nutrients without overloading on any single type. This approach can prevent nutrient deficiencies and support long-term health goals.

Lastly, practical tips for integrating superfoods include keeping a well-stocked pantry and fridge. Make sure to have a variety of superfoods on hand, so creating nutrient-rich meals is convenient and stress-free. Batch cooking and meal prepping can save time and help maintain balance throughout the week. For example, cooking a large batch of quinoa and roasted vegetables can provide the foundation for several meals.

Creating balanced meal plans with superfoods isn't just about throwing a bunch of "healthy" ingredients together. It's about crafting meals that provide comprehensive nutrition while also being delicious and satisfying. By understanding the nutritional benefits of each superfood and thoughtfully incorporating them into daily meals, it's possible to significantly enhance health and well-being over the long term.

Chapter 21:
Superfoods for Specific Health Goals

Understanding how specific superfoods can target particular health goals is vital for anyone looking to enhance their well-being. For heart health, foods rich in omega-3 fatty acids, like salmon and flaxseeds, work wonders by reducing inflammation and lowering cholesterol levels. For those aiming to manage their weight, incorporating high-fiber foods like chia seeds and various legumes helps in promoting satiety and reducing overall calorie intake. Furthermore, superfoods such as blueberries and broccoli are packed with antioxidants essential for brain health, potentially reducing the risk of cognitive decline. By strategically selecting superfoods that align with your unique health goals, you can create a tailored dietary plan that not only nourishes your body but also empowers you to achieve optimal health and longevity efficiently.

Superfoods for Heart Health

Incorporating superfoods into your diet is an excellent way to promote heart health. Foods rich in omega-3 fatty acids, such as salmon and flaxseeds, play a crucial role in reducing inflammation and lowering triglyceride levels, which are important for cardiovascular well-being. Additionally, leafy greens like kale and spinach are powerhouses packed with vitamins, minerals, and antioxidants that help to lower blood pressure and improve arterial function. Nuts, particularly almonds and walnuts, provide a significant source of heart-healthy monounsaturated fats and help to reduce bad cholesterol levels. Whole grains, including quinoa and brown rice, offer fiber that assists in maintaining healthy blood pressure and improving overall heart function. By regularly including these nutrient-dense options in your meals, you can support your cardiovascular system and pave the way to a healthier heart.

Recipes for Heart-Friendly Meals can revolutionize your approach to cardiovascular health by providing delicious and nourishing meal options. With a focus on superfoods known to support heart health, these recipes are crafted to not only taste superb but also to provide the essential nutrients your heart craves. We've combined widely recognized heart-friendly ingredients like leafy greens, whole grains, and healthy oils in various mouth-watering dishes.

First on our list is a **Quinoa and Kale Salad**. Quinoa, often dubbed a super grain, is rich in protein and fiber, crucial for maintaining steady blood sugar levels and keeping your heart in good condition. Kale, lauded for its high levels of vitamins K and C, antioxidants, and fiber, makes an excellent companion to quinoa. Here's how you can whip up this simple, heart-healthy salad:

1 cup of cooked quinoa

2 cups of chopped kale (massage the leaves with a bit of olive oil to soften)

1/2 cup of pomegranate seeds

1/4 cup of chopped almonds

3 tablespoons of olive oil

2 tablespoons of lemon juice

Salt and pepper to taste

Combine all the ingredients in a large bowl, toss well, and serve chilled. This salad is a colorful and nutrient-dense way to keep your heart health in check.

Moving on to a heartier option, the **Lentil and Sweet Potato Stew** offers both warmth and nourishment. Lentils are packed with fiber, while sweet potatoes provide a good supply of vitamins A and C. Both components support a healthy heart by reducing cholesterol and lowering blood pressure. This stew is perfect for a filling and heart-healthy dinner option:

1 cup of green or brown lentils, rinsed

1 large sweet potato, diced

2 carrots, sliced

1 onion, diced

2 garlic cloves, minced

4 cups of vegetable broth

1 teaspoon of turmeric

1 teaspoon of cumin

1/2 teaspoon of black pepper

1 tablespoon of olive oil

In a large pot, heat the olive oil and sauté the onion and garlic until translucent. Add the turmeric, cumin, and black pepper, cooking for another minute. Add the remaining ingredients and bring to a boil. Reduce the heat and let it simmer for about 25-30 minutes, or until the lentils and sweet potatoes are tender. Serve hot with a sprinkle of fresh parsley.

An entrée worth trying is **Salmon with Spinach and Brown Rice**. Salmon is a fantastic source of omega-3 fatty acids, which are vital for heart health. Spinach adds an extra boost of iron, magnesium, and fiber, while brown rice provides the kind of slow-burning energy that benefits heart health. Here's how to prepare this delightful dish:

2 salmon fillets

1 tablespoon of olive oil

4 cups of fresh spinach leaves

1 cup of cooked brown rice

Juice of 1 lemon

Salt and pepper to taste

Preheat your oven to 375°F (190°C). Place the salmon fillets on a baking sheet, drizzle with olive oil and lemon juice, and season with salt and pepper. Bake for about 15-20 minutes, or until the salmon flakes easily with a fork. In a pan, sauté the spinach with a bit of olive oil until wilted. Serve the salmon on a bed of spinach with a side of brown rice for a balanced, nutrient-packed meal.

For a refreshing side, try the **Berry and Avocado Salad**. Berries like strawberries and raspberries are loaded with antioxidants and vitamins, while avocados provide a healthy dose of monounsaturated fats, key for reducing bad cholesterol levels. This salad is as delicious as it is nourishing:

1 cup of fresh strawberries, sliced

1 cup of fresh raspberries

1 avocado, diced

4 cups of mixed greens (such as arugula and spinach)

2 tablespoons of olive oil

1 tablespoon of balsamic vinegar

Salt and pepper to taste

In a large salad bowl, combine the strawberries, raspberries, avocado, and mixed greens. Whisk together the olive oil, balsamic vinegar, salt, and pepper in a small bowl, then drizzle over the salad. Toss gently to combine and enjoy this invigorating side dish, which can also serve as a light main course.

Don't forget about snacks—healthy nibbling can be part of a heart-friendly diet. **Almond and Dark Chocolate Trail Mix** is an excellent choice. Almonds are rich in healthy fats, fiber, and protein, which can help improve cholesterol levels. Dark chocolate, when eaten in moderation, can provide antioxidants that benefit the heart. Here's your go-to recipe for this trail mix:

1 cup of raw almonds

1/2 cup of unsweetened dark chocolate chips

1/2 cup of dried cranberries (make sure they have no added sugar)

1/4 cup of pumpkin seeds

Mix all the ingredients in a large container and portion out individual servings. This trail mix is perfect for a grab-and-go snack that contributes to heart health without compromising on flavor.

A warm, comforting breakfast that's beneficial to your heart is an essential part of any healthy eating plan. **Oatmeal with Chia Seeds and Berries** combines the soluble fiber from oats and chia seeds to help lower cholesterol. Berries add a burst of vitamins and antioxidants:

1 cup of rolled oats

2 tablespoons of chia seeds

2 cups of water or milk of choice

1/2 cup of mixed berries

1 tablespoon of honey or maple syrup

1/2 teaspoon of ground cinnamon

In a pot, bring the water or milk to a boil. Add the rolled oats and chia seeds, then reduce heat to simmer for about 10-15 minutes, stirring occasionally.

Superfoods for Weight Management

For those looking to maintain or lose weight, incorporating superfoods into your diet can be a game-changer. Superfoods like chia seeds, quinoa, and leafy greens are not only packed with essential nutrients but also help in keeping you full for longer periods due to their high fiber content. This feeling of satiety can assist in reducing overall calorie intake without leaving you feeling deprived. Additionally, the thermogenic properties of certain superfoods, such as green tea and chili peppers, can boost your metabolism, aiding in more effective calorie-burning. Including these nutrient-rich foods regularly in your meals can provide a sustainable and healthful approach to weight management.

Tips and Meal Ideas for Weight Control Superfoods play a vital role in weight control and management. Incorporating these nutrient-dense foods into your daily diet can help you feel full, reduce cravings, and provide the essential nutrients your body needs to stay healthy. Here are some practical tips and meal ideas tailored for weight control using various superfoods discussed in this book.

The cornerstone of weight control is portion control. Opting for superfoods such as leafy greens, berries, and lean proteins can naturally help you manage portion sizes while delivering high satiety. For instance, start your meals with a leafy green salad that includes kale or spinach. These greens are incredibly nutrient-dense and low in calories, helping you feel full without adding extra pounds.

Breakfast is a critical meal for weight control. Oat-based breakfasts fortified with chia seeds and berries can be incredibly satisfying. A simple example is overnight oats mixed with chia seeds and topped with fresh blueberries and raspberries. These ingredients are rich in fiber and antioxidants, which not only promote digestive health but also help control hunger pangs throughout the day.

When it comes to snacks, choosing nutrient-dense options like nuts and seeds can make a big difference. Almonds are a fantastic option. Try making your own trail mix with almonds, pumpkin seeds, and dried goji berries for a snack that's both portable and filling. This provides a balanced mix of protein, healthy fats, and fiber, making it easier to avoid reaching for less healthy options.

If you find yourself craving something sweet, smoothies can be incredibly versatile and satisfying. Create a green smoothie with a base of unsweetened almond milk, a handful of spinach, half a banana, and a tablespoon of chia seeds. Add a quarter cup of frozen strawberries or blueberries. This type of smoothie is not only refreshing but also low in calories and high in essential nutrients and fiber.

Lunch and dinner options can be just as satisfying when crafted with superfoods. A quinoa salad mixed with a variety of colorful vegetables like bell peppers, cucumbers, and parsley can be both filling and nutritious. Topped with a dressing made from olive oil and lemon juice, this dish is low in calories but packed with flavor and nutrients. The high fiber content in quinoa also aids in making you feel full longer.

Proteins are essential for weight control, and lean options like salmon or lentils can be particularly beneficial. Consider a dinner of grilled salmon seasoned with turmeric and served with a side of steamed broccoli. Both salmon and broccoli contain properties that promote heart health and aid in weight management. Additionally, lentil soup, which is high in protein and fiber, can be a hearty addition to your meal plan. Lentils provide long-lasting energy, which can help reduce overeating.

Experimenting with fermented foods can also contribute to weight control. Foods like kefir and kimchi are rich in probiotics, which promote a healthy gut microbiome—a key factor in maintaining a balanced weight. Incorporate kefir into your breakfast smoothies or as a base for salad dressings. Kimchi can be a spicy, flavorful addition to many dishes, adding both zest and health benefits.

Cooking methods matter as well. Instead of frying, opt for steaming, grilling, or baking your foods. For example, baking sweet potatoes rather than frying them preserves their nutritional value and reduces unnecessary calorie intake. Sweet potatoes are high in fiber and can be used in various dishes, from sweet potato fries to nutritious soups.

Integrating more whole grains into your diet is another effective strategy. Whole grains like brown rice and quinoa contain more fiber than their refined counterparts, helping you feel fuller faster. For lunch, consider making a brown rice bowl filled with an assortment of vegetables, lean protein like tofu or chicken, and a sprinkle of seeds or nuts for added crunch and nutrients.

Spices can also be impactful. Spices such as cayenne pepper, garlic, and ginger can boost metabolism and add flavor to your meals without the need for extra salt or sugar. A turmeric and ginger tea, consumed in the afternoon or evening, can have anti-inflammatory benefits and help regulate appetite.

Don't forget about beverages. Replacing sugary drinks with herbal teas and water can significantly reduce calorie intake. Green tea is particularly beneficial because of its antioxidant properties and metabolism-boosting capabilities. Sip on green tea throughout the day to help stay hydrated and full.

Finally, planning and prepping your meals in advance can significantly aid in weight control. Pre-cook items like quinoa, brown rice, and boiled eggs at the beginning of the week. Store them in portion-controlled containers, and you'll have easy, ready-to-eat components for balanced meals throughout the week. Incorporate a variety of superfoods into your weekly menu to keep your meals interesting and nutritious.

In conclusion, weight control involves making mindful choices and creating balanced meals that are rich in nutrient-dense superfoods. By incorporating leafy greens, whole grains, lean proteins, nuts, seeds, and fermented foods into your diet, you can enjoy flavorful and satisfying meals while managing your weight effectively. With a bit of planning and creativity, superfoods can become the cornerstone of a healthy and balanced lifestyle.

Chapter 22:
Seasonal Superfoods

Embracing the rhythm of the seasons can be transformative for your health, as each time of year brings its own bounty of nutrient-packed superfoods. In winter, indulge in hearty root vegetables like sweet potatoes and beets, which are packed with antioxidants and can nourish you from the inside out. As the weather warms, look to vibrant summer produce like berries and tomatoes that burst with vitamins and revitalize your plate. Consuming superfoods at their peak harvest not only maximizes their nutritional value but also supports local agriculture and sustainability efforts. By staying attuned to what each season has to offer, you ensure a varied and balanced diet that can invigorate your journey toward better health and longevity.

winter superfoods

During the chilly winter months, our bodies crave warmth and nourishment from hearty, nutrient-dense foods that support our immune systems and overall well-being. Winter superfoods like root vegetables, dark leafy greens, and citrus fruits are packed with vitamins, minerals, and antioxidants essential for staying healthy when temperatures drop. Beets, for instance, are rich in betalains and fiber, making them excellent for detoxification and digestion. Kale and Swiss chard become even sweeter after a frost, providing a rich source of vitamins A, C, and K, as well as folate. Citrus fruits such as oranges and grapefruits offer a refreshing burst of vitamin C, crucial for immune support. Embracing these winter superfoods not only helps fight off seasonal ailments but also ensures you receive a diverse array of nutrients, promoting longevity and vitality during the coldest time of year.

Recipes Featuring Winter's Best are a celebration of the season's most nutrient-rich superfoods. Winter, often associated with shorter days and chilly weather, brings a unique collection of fruits, vegetables, and spices that can nourish and revitalize the body. The trick to thriving during the colder months lies in incorporating these powerful ingredients into your meals, ensuring every bite supports your health and wellbeing.

Winter superfoods boast an impressive array of vitamins, minerals, and antioxidants, all of which are crucial for maintaining good health. Among them, root vegetables like sweet potatoes and carrots are packed with beta-carotene, while cruciferous vegetables like Brussels sprouts and broccoli provide sulforaphane, a potent antioxidant. Pair these with hearty, warming spices like turmeric and ginger, and you have a recipe lineup that's comforting and beneficial.

Let's start with a simple, yet incredibly nutritious recipe: **Roasted Root Vegetable Medley**. This dish features sweet potatoes, carrots, and parsnips, all seasoned with olive oil, garlic, and rosemary. The roasting process caramelizes the natural sugars in the vegetables, enhancing their flavor and guaranteeing a crowd-pleaser at any table.

Select medium-sized sweet potatoes and parsnips. Peel and cut them into uniform chunks. Toss them in a large mixing bowl with peeled and sliced carrots, a generous drizzle of olive oil, minced garlic, and fresh rosemary sprigs. Spread them out on a baking sheet in a single layer, ensuring they roast evenly. Bake at 400°F (200°C) for about 35-40 minutes, or until they're golden and tender. Season with salt and pepper to taste and serve hot.

Another winter favorite is **Broccoli and Cheddar Soup**. This creamy, satisfying soup marries the vitamin-packed goodness of broccoli with the comforting richness of cheddar cheese. Start by sautéing diced onions in a large pot until they're translucent. Add minced garlic and cook for another minute. Pour in vegetable broth and bring to a simmer before adding chopped broccoli florets. Cook until the broccoli is tender, then blend the mixture until smooth. Return to the pot, stir in shredded cheddar cheese, and season with salt, pepper, and a pinch of nutmeg. Serve warm with a slice of whole grain bread.

Don't overlook the role of spices in boosting both flavor and health benefits. *Turmeric* and *ginger* are particularly effective in winter dishes. Consider a **Golden Milk Turmeric Latte** to start your day on a healthful note. Warm almond milk in a saucepan and whisk in ground turmeric, ground ginger, and a bit of black pepper to enhance absorption. Sweeten with honey or maple syrup to taste and serve warm. This cozy drink not only warms you up but also provides anti-inflammatory and antioxidant benefits.

For a dish that's both exotic and approachable, try **Moroccan-Spiced Carrot and Lentil Soup**. In a large pot, heat olive oil and sauté chopped onions, garlic, and fresh ginger until fragrant. Add ground cumin, coriander, and cinnamon, stirring until the spices are well mixed. Incorporate chopped carrots, red lentils, and vegetable broth. Simmer until the carrots and lentils are tender, then blend partially to create a thick, hearty texture. Finish with a squeeze of fresh lemon juice and finely chopped cilantro.

If you're seeking a satisfying main course, **Winter Greens and Quinoa Salad** offers a fantastic balance of flavors and nutrients. Use a mix of kale and Swiss chard, both rich in vitamins A, C, and K. Cook quinoa according to package instructions and let it cool. Meanwhile, massage the kale and chard leaves with a bit of olive oil to soften them.

Combine the cooked quinoa with the greens, add segments of fresh oranges for a citrusy touch, and sprinkle with pomegranate seeds for an antioxidant boost. Dress the salad with a light vinaigrette made from olive oil, balsamic vinegar, Dijon mustard, and a touch of honey.

Remember, winter produce isn't just about vegetables. Citrus fruits like oranges and grapefruits are in their prime during these months, bringing a burst of color and vitamin C to your meals. A refreshing **Citrus and Fennel Salad** combines the crisp, slightly sweet fennel with juicy orange segments and a simple dressing of olive oil and white wine vinegar. It's a delightful side dish or light lunch that's both invigorating and nourishing.

The benefits of incorporating these winter superfoods into your diet extend beyond immediate nutrition. Roots like sweet potatoes are complex carbohydrates that provide sustained energy, while cruciferous vegetables like broccoli support detoxification processes in the body. Foods rich in antioxidants, such as pomegranates and oranges, help combat oxidative stress and support a healthy immune system, crucial during the flu season.

Winter also calls for some comforting foods. Experiment with a warming bowl of **Spiced Apple and Quinoa Porridge**. Combine quinoa, diced apples, almond milk, and a dash of cinnamon in a pot. Bring to a boil, then reduce the heat and let it simmer until the quinoa is fully cooked and the apples are tender. Sweeten with a bit of maple syrup and top with chopped walnuts or almonds for an extra crunch and nutrient boost.

If ending your meal on a sweet note sounds appealing, consider **Dark Chocolate and Walnut Brownies**. These treats incorporate the antioxidant properties of dark chocolate with the omega-3 benefits of walnuts. Melt high-quality dark chocolate with a touch of coconut oil. In another bowl, mix whole wheat flour, cocoa powder, and a pinch of salt. Beat together eggs and a natural sweetener like agave syrup or coconut sugar, then combine with the melted chocolate. Fold in the dry ingredients and chopped walnuts. Bake at 350°F (175°C) until set but still slightly gooey in the center. These brownies manage to be indulgent yet healthful, proving that healthy eating doesn't mean giving up dessert.

Ultimately, these recipes featuring winter's best not only provide nourishment but also comfort and warmth, making the most of what the season has to offer. By incorporating these nutrient-dense superfoods into your meals, you'll be supporting your body's health and longevity, keeping you vibrant and energized all winter long.

Summer Superfoods

Summer is the perfect season to indulge in vibrant, nutrient-rich superfoods that can enhance your health and vitality. Fresh, locally grown produce like tomatoes, strawberries, and leafy greens are at their peak, packed with antioxidants, vitamins, and minerals that support overall well-being. Watermelon, for example, not only hydrates but also provides a rich source of lycopene, known for its heart-protective benefits. Blueberries, another summer favorite, are famed for their potent antioxidant properties, which combat oxidative stress and promote healthy aging. Incorporating these seasonal superfoods into your meals is a simple, delicious way to boost your nutrient intake and enjoy the unique flavors of summer. Whether it's a refreshing salad, a smoothie bursting with berries, or a light, grilled vegetable dish, the possibilities are endless for creating mouth-watering, health-enhancing summer recipes.

Dishes to Celebrate Summer are more than just an excuse to fire up the barbecue and spend more time outdoors; they're a great opportunity to incorporate nutrient-dense superfoods that can truly elevate your health. Summer's bounty includes a variety of fresh fruits, vegetables, and other superfoods that are at their peak flavor and nutrition, making it the perfect time to get creative in the kitchen. In this section, we're diving into a selection of the finest and most enjoyable summer dishes that highlight these ingredients.

To start, let's talk about one of the season's quintessential ingredients: tomatoes. There is nothing quite like the taste of tomatoes ripened under the summer sun. They are packed with lycopene, which is a powerful antioxidant known to support heart health and reduce the risk of certain cancers. A simple way to enjoy tomatoes is in a Caprese salad. Just layer slices of fresh tomatoes with mozzarella cheese, basil leaves, and drizzle with a bit of olive oil and balsamic vinegar. This dish not only bursts with color and flavor but also brings a host of nutritional benefits.

Next up, think about including an assortment of berries in your summer meals. Strawberries, blueberries, and raspberries are not only deliciously sweet but also rich in vitamins, fiber, and antioxidants. You could prepare a refreshing summer berry salad by mixing these berries with a handful of fresh mint and a sprinkle of lemon zest. This salad can be enjoyed on its own or as a topping for Greek yogurt or oatmeal.

Summer is also the perfect time to indulge in fresh corn. Corn is a versatile superfood that provides vitamins, minerals, and a good amount of fiber. One of the simplest yet most delightful ways to enjoy it is by grilling it on the cob. After it's cooked to smoky, charred perfection, rub it with a little bit of olive oil and sprinkle with chili powder and a squeeze of lime juice. This delicious combination is both satisfying and nourishing.

Let's not forget about leafy greens, which are abundant in the summer months. Spinach, kale, and arugula can be used to whip up nutritious salads and smoothies. For a light and refreshing salad, try mixing baby spinach with sliced strawberries, almonds, and a touch of feta cheese. Toss with a zesty lemon vinaigrette, and you have a meal that is as tasty as it is nutritious.

Avocados reach their peak in summer, making it an ideal time to enjoy their creamy goodness. Rich in healthy fats, fiber, and an array of vitamins, avocados are a versatile superfood that can be used in a plethora of summer dishes. Try making a classic guacamole by mashing avocados and mixing in chopped tomatoes, onions, cilantro, lime juice, and a pinch of salt. Serve with whole grain crackers or veggie sticks for a healthy snack or appetizer.

For those steamy summer evenings when you want something light but satisfying, consider a quinoa and black bean salad. Quinoa is a complete protein and incredibly versatile. Combine cooked quinoa with black beans, chopped bell peppers, corn, red onions, and cilantro. Dress it with a lime-cumin vinaigrette for a dish that's bursting with flavor and nutrition.

Summer isn't complete without some hydrating treats, and watermelon fits the bill perfectly. This juicy fruit is more than just water and sweetness; it's also packed with vitamins A, C, and antioxidants. One creative way to enjoy watermelon is in a savory salad. Mix cubed watermelon with crumbled feta cheese, sliced red onions, and fresh mint leaves. Drizzle with a bit of balsamic reduction for a dish that is equally stunning and refreshing.

Let's talk about seafood. Summer is an excellent time to embrace omega-3-rich fish like salmon. Grilling salmon on a cedar plank imparts a smoky flavor that pairs beautifully with a fresh mango salsa. Simply dice mangoes, red bell peppers, red onions, and jalapenos. Mix with a bit of lime juice and cilantro for a tangy and sweet accompaniment to your perfectly grilled fish. This balanced meal is not only delicious but also promotes heart health and overall well-being.

For dessert, berries with Greek yogurt are a simple but delectable choice that's packed with protein, probiotics, and antioxidants. Layer a mix of raspberries, blueberries, and strawberries over a bowl of creamy

Greek yogurt. Top it off with a drizzle of honey and a handful of granola for some crunch. This dessert is not only satisfying and delicious but also supports gut health and provides lasting energy.

Chilled soups are a delightful way to start a summer meal. Gazpacho, a cold Spanish soup made from blended tomatoes, cucumbers, bell peppers, onions, and garlic, is a refreshing appetizer that's brimming with nutrients. Serve it chilled with a sprinkle of fresh herbs such as basil or cilantro. This no-cook dish is a fantastic way to beat the heat while packing in a variety of vitamins and antioxidants.

Incorporating summer superfoods into your meals doesn't have to be complicated. It can be as simple as making smoothies using seasonal fruits, nuts, and seeds. Create a vibrant green smoothie by blending baby spinach, frozen mango, avocado, chia seeds, and almond milk. This nutrient-dense drink is a perfect way to kickstart your day or recharge after a workout.

The versatility of superfoods allows you to experiment and customize according to your tastes. For your summer barbecues, try marinating chicken breasts in a mixture of olive oil, lemon juice, garlic, and fresh herbs like rosemary and thyme. Grill to perfection and serve alongside a zesty cucumber-tomato salad. This combo not only promises great flavor but also ensures a healthy and balanced meal.

And let's not underestimate the power of fresh herbs. Basil, mint, cilantro, and parsley are at their peak in summer. They can elevate any dish, adding not only flavor but also a burst of nutrients. A pesto made from fresh basil, pine nuts, garlic, and olive oil can transform simple grilled vegetables or pasta into a gourmet experience.

So, whether you're hosting a backyard barbecue or enjoying a quiet dinner on the patio, summer offers endless opportunities to celebrate with nutritious and flavorful dishes. By focusing on a variety of fresh, seasonal superfoods, you can create meals that not only taste amazing but also support your overall health and longevity. Enjoy the bounty of the season, and don't be afraid to get creative in your kitchen.

Chapter 23:
Integrating Superfoods in Daily Life

Seamlessly incorporating superfoods into your daily routine may seem daunting at first, but with a few simple strategies, it can become second nature. Start by adding a handful of antioxidant-rich berries to your morning oatmeal or smoothie, infusing your day with vital nutrients from the get-go. When meal prepping, consider swapping out regular grains with quinoa or brown rice to boost your fiber intake, promoting digestive health and sustained energy levels throughout the day. Snacks can be as straightforward as a small serving of chia pudding or a few almonds, each packed with essential vitamins and minerals. To make it fun for kids, sneak superfoods into their meals by blending spinach into sauces or baking with nutrient-dense flours. Consistently opting for olive oil as your primary cooking fat instead of conventional oils can bolster heart health while enhancing the flavor of your dishes. By gradually integrating these nutrient-dense foods into your meals, you're not just adopting a healthier lifestyle but also ensuring longevity and sustained vitality.

Quick and Easy Superfood Snacks

Incorporating superfoods into your day doesn't have to be complicated or time-consuming. For those hectic moments when you need a quick nutritional boost, try snacking on simple yet powerful options like a handful of goji berries, a cup of antioxidant-rich blueberries, or a blend of nuts and seeds such as almonds and chia seeds. These snacks not only pack a punch with their high nutrient content but are also conveniently portable, making them perfect for busy days. You can elevate your snack game by preparing easy recipes like chia pudding topped with fresh fruit, or kale chips seasoned with a pinch of sea salt. With these quick and easy superfood snacks, you'll find it effortless to fuel your body with the nutrients it needs, enhancing your health and longevity even in the busiest moments.

Snack Ideas for Busy Days When you're juggling a packed schedule, it's easy to fall into the trap of reaching for unhealthy snacks. But the good news is, with a little planning, you can have nutrient-dense superfood snacks that keep you energized and focused throughout the day. It's not about deprivation; it's about making smarter choices that fuel your body and support your long-term health goals.

One quick and simple option is a smoothie. Pre-packaged smoothies from the store often contain added sugars and preservatives, but making your own can be a game-changer. Using a base like unsweetened almond milk or coconut water, toss in a handful of spinach, a cup of mixed berries, a tablespoon of chia seeds, and half an avocado. Blend until smooth, and you have a nutrient-packed snack that's ready to go.

If you're in the mood for something crunchy, homemade trail mix is an excellent option. Store-bought varieties can be laden with sodium and sugar, but creating your own allows you to control the ingredients. Mix together raw almonds, pumpkin seeds, dried goji berries, and dark chocolate chunks. Not only is it tasty, but it also provides a balanced mix of protein, healthy fats, and antioxidants.

For those days when you're constantly on the move, energy balls are lifesavers. These bite-sized snacks are easy to prepare and store well. Combine oats, almond butter, chia seeds, and a touch of honey in a food processor. Roll into small balls and refrigerate. These can be customized with add-ins like cacao nibs or dried cranberries for an additional nutrient boost.

Another savory option is roasted chickpeas. High in protein and fiber, chickpeas are incredibly satisfying. To make, drain and rinse a can of chickpeas, then toss them in olive oil and your favorite spices like paprika and garlic powder. Roast in the oven until crispy and golden. These can be stored in an airtight container, making them perfect for on-the-go snacking.

Vegetable sticks paired with a nutrient-rich dip can also be a refreshing snack. Cut up carrots, celery, and bell peppers, and serve them with a homemade hummus or a creamy avocado dip. Hummus is not only delicious but also provides a good source of protein and fiber, especially if made from chickpeas and tahini. An avocado dip can add healthy fats and vitamins to your snack routine.

Speaking of avocado, don't forget about avocado toast. Using whole grain bread, mash half an avocado and spread it on the toast. Sprinkle with chia seeds, flaxseeds, or a dash of turmeric for an extra superfood punch. It's a simple yet satisfying snack that can keep you full for hours.

For a protein-packed snack that requires no preparation, consider Greek yogurt with a handful of berries and a sprinkle of flaxseeds. Greek yogurt is an excellent source of calcium and probiotics, while the berries provide antioxidants and the flaxseeds add essential omega-3 fatty acids. This combination is perfect for boosting your immune system and maintaining good gut health.

Nori sheets are another portable and nutrient-dense snack. These seaweed snacks are crunchy, savory, and packed with minerals like iodine, which is essential for thyroid function. You can find pre-packaged nori snacks or make your own at home by brushing nori sheets with a bit of sesame oil and baking them until crisp.

When the sweet tooth hits, reaching for dark chocolate can be a healthy choice. Look for high-quality dark chocolate with at least 70% cacao content, which ensures you get more antioxidants and less sugar. Combining a small piece of dark chocolate with a handful of nuts, like almonds or walnuts, can make for a satisfying and wholesome snack.

Edamame, or young soybeans, are another excellent, easy-to-prepare snack. Simply boil or steam them and sprinkle a bit of sea salt on top. These are high in protein and fiber, making them ideal for sustaining energy levels throughout your busy day. Plus, they're fun to eat and can be a great way to keep your hands busy if you're trying to avoid less healthy snacks.

If you're looking for a more substantial snack that could double as a light meal, consider whole grain wraps. Use a whole grain tortilla, spread a layer of hummus or nut butter, and fill it with sliced vegetables like cucumbers, bell peppers, and shredded carrots. Roll it up and cut it into bite-sized pieces for a convenient, nutrient-dense option.

Incorporating snacks like these into your daily routine can significantly improve your overall nutritional intake without much extra effort. Swapping out processed snacks for whole, nutrient-rich superfoods will provide your body with the essential vitamins, minerals, and antioxidants it needs to thrive. Over time, you'll likely notice increased energy levels, better digestion, and an overall improvement in well-being.

Preparing these snacks ahead of time can also streamline your busy days. Set aside a small block of time each week to prep your snacks and store them in individual containers. This makes it easy to grab something nutritious when you're short on time and prevents the temptation of reaching for less healthy options.

Incorporating superfood snacks into your hectic lifestyle might seem challenging, but with a bit of planning, it becomes second nature. Try different combinations and experiment with flavors to keep your snacks interesting and enjoyable. You'll be amazed at how making small, consistent changes can lead to significant improvements in your health and longevity.

Superfoods for Kids

Integrating superfoods into your child's diet doesn't have to be a struggle. By creatively incorporating nutrient-rich foods like blueberries, spinach, and quinoa, you can turn everyday meals into power-packed experiences. Think of colorful smoothie bowls topped with chia seeds and fresh berries or mini veggie muffins sneaking in kale and carrots. The key is making the dishes fun and visually appealing while ensuring they deliver essential vitamins and minerals. Remember, the earlier children develop a taste for these wholesome foods, the more likely they'll maintain healthy eating habits into adulthood. With a bit of ingenuity, you can make superfood-filled meals both enjoyable and nutritious for your little ones.

Making Nutritious Meals Fun hinges on the intersection of creativity and health, particularly when it comes to feeding kids. Integrating nutrient-rich superfoods into meals that children will actually eat and enjoy can sometimes feel like a Herculean task. But it doesn't have to be a constant battle of wills. The trick lies in making the meals engaging, colorful, and aligned with their taste buds. So, let's explore ways to turn those healthy ingredients into exciting dishes that even the pickiest eaters would love.

One effective strategy is to involve kids in the meal preparation process. When they have a hand in making their food, they're more likely to try it. You can start with cooking classes in your own kitchen. Teach them to make colorful smoothie bowls with a rainbow of fruits like blueberries, strawberries, and bananas, topped with a sprinkle of chia seeds. Not only does this make for a nutrient-packed breakfast or snack, but it also turns eating into an art project full of vibrant colors and varied textures.

Another way to make nutritious meals fun is through themed meals. Kids love themes, whether it's for a birthday party or a casual weeknight dinner. Create a "Superhero Meal" using superfoods that contribute to their "superpowers." Spinach for strength like Popeye, sweet potatoes for energy like the Flash, and berries for a sharp mind like a high-tech genius. Presenting these foods within a theme can make them more exciting and relatable.

Bento boxes offer another fantastic way to make meals visually appealing. These compartmentalized lunchboxes allow you to include a variety of colorful foods that kids can pick and choose from. For example, fill the different sections with sliced veggies, nuts, fruit, and a whole grain snack. Add a small container of hummus or a yogurt dip to complete the meal. The visual appeal of a well-organized Bento box encourages kids to try a little bit of everything. Plus, the bite-sized portions can make unfamiliar foods seem less intimidating.

Don't underestimate the power of shapes and sizes when making food fun for kids. Simple tools like cookie cutters can transform ordinary sandwiches, fruits, and veggies into stars, hearts, and even animals. Think about making star-shaped cucumber slices, heart-shaped carrot coins, or sandwiches in the shape of dinosaurs. These small touches can go a long way in making the meal more enticing.

Moreover, incorporating storytelling can turn a meal into an adventure. Tell a story about where the superfood comes from and how it got its superpowers. For instance, explain how ancient warriors ate quinoa to boost their energy before battles, or how explorers relied on hearty lentil stews during their journeys. This not only captivates children's imaginations but also provides them with an educational background on the nutritious foods they're eating.

For special occasions or just to break the monotony, holding a "Build Your Own" event can be incredibly engaging. Let kids build their own salads, tacos, or pizzas using a variety of healthy ingredients. Provide a selection of toppings, spreads, and dressings made from nutrient-dense superfoods. Kids will have a blast creating their perfect meal, and they might even be more willing to try new ingredients in the process.

Creative plating is another method to make nutritious meals appealing. Arrange foods to create images or patterns, such as a butterfly using slices of bell peppers for wings and a baby carrot for the body. Food art not only looks cool but can also make the meal feel special. This method can transform even the most mundane veggies into a visual feast.

Encouragement through positive reinforcement can also work wonders. Praise their choices and willingness to try new foods, even if they don't love everything right away. Building a positive association with healthy eating sets the stage for long-term habits. Young minds are impressionable, and your enthusiasm for nutritious foods can ignite their interest.

If your children have a favorite dish that isn't typically healthy, try making a nutritious version. For example, if they love mac and cheese, consider using whole grain pasta and incorporating pureed butternut squash into the cheese sauce. Not only does it add nutrients, but it also doesn't drastically change the flavor, making it a subtle yet effective way to improve the dish's nutritional profile.

Remember snacks shouldn't be an afterthought. Start considering them as mini-meals that contribute to your children's overall nutrient intake. Smoothies, energy balls, and veggie sticks with fun dips like guacamole or Greek yogurt-based spreads can turn snack time into an opportunity for boosting their daily fruit and vegetable quota.

Storybooks and cartoons featuring healthy foods can subtly influence kids to develop a liking towards those foods. If a beloved character enjoys a specific superfood, your child might be more inclined to give it a try. Search for books that celebrate healthy eating, turning it from a mundane task into an exciting adventure.

Lastly, never underestimate the power of setting a good example. Children often model the behaviors they see in adults. Show enthusiasm for nutritious foods and make a point to enjoy them yourself. Share the reasons why you appreciate these foods, whether it's for their taste or the way they make you feel. It's not just about telling them to eat their greens – it's about showing them how you enjoy eating yours.

In conclusion, making nutritious meals fun is an exercise in creativity, storytelling, and engaging the senses. By gradually incorporating these methods, you're not only enhancing their current diet but setting them up with lifelong healthy eating habits. It's about transforming the perception of nutrient-dense foods from something they "have to" eat into something they "want to" eat, all while keeping it enjoyable and visually appealing.

Chapter 24:
Superfood Myths and Truths

The term "superfood" often evokes images of exotic, miraculous foods, but it's important to separate fact from fiction. While many superfoods like blueberries and kale truly offer impressive nutrient profiles, others may not live up to the hype. For example, some people believe that consuming a single superfood can dramatically transform their health overnight, when in reality, long-term health benefits come from a balanced diet and consistent lifestyle habits. It's crucial to understand that no one food possesses a magical cure-all property. Integrating a variety of nutrient-dense foods into your daily diet is the real key to harnessing their potential benefits. Myths, such as superfoods needing to be expensive or hard to find, also need debunking; many everyday items like legumes and whole grains offer remarkable advantages. Understanding these truths empowers you to make informed choices and truly benefit from what superfoods have to offer.

Debunking Common Myths

When it comes to superfoods, misconceptions abound, often leading to confusion about their true benefits. One prevalent myth is that superfoods alone can compensate for an otherwise unhealthy diet. While nutrient-dense foods like kale, blueberries, and quinoa are packed with vitamins and antioxidants, they are not magic bullets. Another common fallacy is believing that all exotic and expensive superfoods are superior to local produce. In reality, everyday items like spinach and oats can be just as potent in delivering essential nutrients. It's also worth noting that simply adding a superfood to your diet won't yield immediate health results; consistent, balanced nutrition—integrated with an overall healthy lifestyle—is key. By debunking these myths, we aim to provide a clearer, more practical approach to incorporating superfoods effectively.

Clarifying Superfood Misconceptions is essential in navigating the sometimes muddled world of nutrient-dense foods. With so much information floating around, it's easy to get lost or misled by flashy marketing claims or outdated beliefs. Our goal is to demystify superfoods, separating facts from fiction so you can make informed decisions about what ends up on your plate.

One common misconception is that superfoods are a modern invention. While the term itself may be relatively new, many superfoods have been staples in various cultures for thousands of years. For example, quinoa was a sacred grain of the Incas, and pomegranates have been cherished since ancient Persian times. These foods' potent benefits aren't a recent discovery but rather a rediscovery in the context of modern nutritional science.

Another myth is that superfoods must be exotic or hard to find. While acai berries and goji berries often steal the spotlight, many superfoods are likely already in your pantry or grocery store. Think blueberries, spinach, almonds, and green tea. These accessible items are just as nutrient-rich and can easily be integrated into your daily routine without breaking the bank.

There's also a misconception that superfoods are a cure-all. No single food can magically erase health problems; instead, it's about incorporating a variety of nutrient-dense foods into a balanced diet. Superfoods work best as part of a holistic approach to health, one that includes regular physical activity, adequate sleep, and stress management. Over-relying on a single type of food for all your nutritional needs isn't just unrealistic; it can also be unhealthy.

Some believe that the nutritional value of superfoods diminishes through cooking or processing. While it's true that some vitamins and antioxidants degrade with heat, many superfoods are incredibly versatile and retain most of their benefits. For example, cooked tomatoes are richer in the antioxidant lycopene than raw ones. The key is knowing which preparation methods enhance certain nutrients and which protect them.

Equally important to clarify is the misunderstanding that all superfoods are expensive. Yes, some superfoods can have higher price tags, particularly when marketed and packaged as specialty items. However, bulk bin sections and local farmer's markets often offer more budget-friendly options. Staples like lentils, oats, and brown rice are cost-effective and pack a nutritional punch. Remember, a superfood's value isn't just in its nutrient profile but also in how accessible and sustainable it is for your lifestyle.

A related misconception is the notion that you need to consume large quantities of superfoods to reap their benefits. In reality, even small amounts can make a significant difference. For instance, a tablespoon of chia seeds or a handful of walnuts can provide a substantial dose of omega-3 fatty acids and fiber. It's not about eating tons but rather about consistently incorporating them into your diet day by day.

There is also a tendency to assume that the newest superfood trend is superior to traditional whole foods. This usually isn't the case. The nutritional industry is rife with trends that ebb and flow. While novel superfoods can add variety and unique benefits to your diet, they shouldn't overshadow the foundational foods like fruits, vegetables, whole grains, and lean proteins that have stood the test of time.

Contrary to popular belief, superfoods don't need to be consumed raw to be effective. Though eating raw can preserve certain nutrients, it's not a prerequisite for health benefits. Many superfoods release more nutrients when cooked or fermented. For example, fermenting soybeans into tempeh enhances their digestibility and nutritional value. Diversifying your preparation methods can maximize the benefits you get from these potent foods.

Another persistent myth is that synthetic supplements can replace whole superfoods. While supplements can help fill nutritional gaps, they often lack the complex mix of nutrients and fiber found in whole foods. The synergy of vitamins, minerals, antioxidants, and other compounds in whole foods can't be easily replicated in a pill. Prioritizing whole superfoods ensures you're getting the most comprehensive nutritional benefits.

Lastly, it's common to think that superfoods are just about physical health. Though their benefits for physical wellness are well-documented, many superfoods have profound effects on mental health too. Turmeric, for example, is renowned not only for its anti-inflammatory properties but also for its potential to improve mood and alleviate symptoms of depression. Integrating superfoods into your diet can thus support a more balanced mind and body.

Clearing up these misconceptions is a step toward a more informed and empowered approach to nutrition. By shedding light on the facts and debunking these myths, we hope you'll find it easier to make choices that truly benefit your health and longevity. There's no need for confusion—just a commitment to understanding and appreciating the real, multifaceted power of superfoods.

In the chapters to come, we will continue to provide practical tips, science-backed insights, and delicious recipes. These will not only help you integrate superfoods into your daily life but also help you navigate the often overwhelming world of nutrition with clarity and confidence. With the right knowledge, superfoods can become a seamless and enriching part of your journey towards a healthier, longer life.

Verified Benefits of Superfoods

Superfoods are more than just buzzworthy; they're backed by substantial scientific evidence demonstrating their profound impact on health and longevity. Rich in vital nutrients like antioxidants, vitamins, minerals, and healthy fats, these foods support a range of bodily functions and protection mechanisms. Regular consumption of superfoods can contribute to improved heart health, enhanced brain function, strengthened immune system, and reduced inflammation. For instance, leafy greens like kale and spinach are packed with iron and calcium, while berries offer an abundance of antioxidants that combat oxidative stress. By integrating a variety of these nutrient-dense foods into your daily diet, you empower your body to function at its optimum level, thereby promoting long-term wellness and vitality.

Understanding True Health Benefits serves as a cornerstone for grasping the genuine advantages of integrating superfoods into our daily lives. At its core, this sub-section aims to dismantle the often murky and confused conversations surrounding superfoods, providing a clear roadmap for those wishing to leverage their full potential for health and longevity. More than just buzzwords or fleeting trends, the true health benefits of superfoods are rooted in centuries of traditional use combined with contemporary scientific validation.

A significant part of understanding these benefits is recognizing that not all superfoods are created equal. Each one brings its own set of unique attributes—from antioxidant capabilities and anti-inflammatory properties to enhanced energy levels and improved digestion. For example, blueberries are known for their rich content of anthocyanins that help combat oxidative stress, while nuts and seeds like almonds and chia are incredible sources of essential fatty acids and proteins that our bodies can't produce on their own. Awareness and intentionality when choosing superfoods are crucial for achieving the desired health outcomes they promise.

Science and tradition often come together to reveal the profound impact these foods can have. Modern research consistently validates what many ancestral diets have known for generations: superfoods are not just a part of a meal; they are powerful tools for maintaining and improving health. For example, turmeric's role as an anti-inflammatory agent has been documented in Ayurveda for centuries, yet it's only recently that Western medicine has caught up to understand curcumin's potential in reducing chronic inflammation and promoting joint health.

Beyond their nutrient profiles, the holistic benefits of superfoods span a broad spectrum. They play a pivotal role in cardiovascular health, aiding in the management of cholesterol levels and reducing the risk of heart disease. Numerous studies link the consumption of certain superfoods to improved heart function, owing to their high levels of beneficial fats and antioxidants. For instance, incorporating foods rich in omega-3 fatty acids like salmon can significantly contribute to heart health by lowering blood pressure and reducing plaque build-up in arteries.

Gut health, too, is profoundly impacted by these nutrient-dense foods. Fermented options like kefir and kombucha introduce beneficial probiotics into the digestive system, establishing a balanced gut flora that supports digestion and enhances the immune function. These microorganisms help break down food more efficiently, ensuring your body absorbs the maximum nutrients from what you consume. Furthermore, maintaining a healthy gut flora can have cascading benefits, affecting everything from mental health to skin clarity.

The anti-inflammatory properties of many superfoods can't be overstated. Inflammation, often considered the root of many chronic diseases, can be mitigated through a diet rich in inflammatory-fighting ingredients. Superfoods such as ginger and turmeric are widely acknowledged for their ability to down-regulate pro-inflammatory genes and decrease levels of inflammatory biomarkers in the body. This not only reduces the risk of chronic diseases but also improves overall well-being and quality of life.

It's essential to mention that the benefits of superfoods extend to mental health as well. Nutrients such as omega-3 fatty acids, found in foods like walnuts and flaxseed, are critical for brain health. These nutrients support cognitive function, improve mood, and can even alleviate symptoms of depression and anxiety. Research has shown that diets rich in omega-3s are associated with lower rates of neurodegenerative diseases like Alzheimer's, providing a compelling case for their inclusion in your diet.

However, the journey to understanding true health benefits isn't solely about the individual components of these foods. It's about how they interact within our unique systems and among themselves when included in a balanced diet. Synergistic effects can occur, where the combined impact of consuming multiple superfoods is greater than the sum of their separate benefits. For example, pairing vitamin C-rich foods like oranges with iron-rich plant-based foods helps enhance iron absorption, effectively combating anemia more efficiently than consuming these nutrients in isolation.

Moreover, consistent consumption is key. The cumulative effects of eating superfoods regularly can lead to long-term health benefits that are often gradual but significant. Unlike immediate results seen from medications, the benefits of superfoods usually manifest over time. This means a daily commitment to incorporating these foods into your meals can yield dividends in the form of prolonged energy levels, improved mental clarity, and a robust immune system.

Educational initiatives play a vital role in disseminating this information. Many people are still unaware of the full spectrum of benefits superfoods offer and how best to incorporate them into their daily routines. Classes, books, and online resources created by nutritionists and health experts can guide individuals in making informed choices. This kind of informed consumerism empowers individuals not just to make healthier food choices but to understand why those choices matter.

An often overlooked aspect is the role superfoods play in preventive medicine. By incorporating them into our diets, we can potentially stave off a multitude of health issues before they require medical intervention. For instance, foods high in fiber like whole grains and legumes help regulate blood sugar levels, playing a critical role in preventing Type 2 diabetes. Similarly, the antioxidants in berries can neutralize free radicals, reducing the risk of developing cancer.

Another layer to understanding true health benefits encompasses how superfoods can improve athletic performance and recovery. Nutrient-rich options like beetroot juice have been shown to enhance endurance by improving oxygen efficiency in muscles. Superfoods also aid in quicker recovery post-exercise due to their anti-inflammatory and muscle-repair properties. For athletes and fitness enthusiasts, this means a diet rich in these foods can lead to more effective, consistent training sessions.

Lastly, it's important to appreciate the emotional and psychological satisfaction that accompanies the consumption of superfoods. Many of these foods are not only nutrient-dense but also delectably flavorful and versatile. The joy of preparing a vibrant, antioxidant-rich smoothie or a hearty quinoa salad can have a positive impact on mental well-being, reinforcing healthy eating habits as a pleasurable, sustainable lifestyle choice.

In summary, understanding the true health benefits of superfoods requires a multifaceted approach, considering their individual and synergistic effects, as well as their role in preventative health and overall well-being. Integrating these nutrient-dense options into your daily diet is not just a trend but a profound step towards longevity and improved quality of life. The insights shared here provide a strong foundation for anyone keen to explore the world of superfoods, offering both scientific and practical perspectives to inform and inspire a healthier future.

Chapter 25:
Sustainable Superfoods

The journey towards a healthier, more vibrant life doesn't stop at the nutritional benefits of superfoods—it extends to how these nutrient-dense foods are cultivated and consumed sustainably. Incorporating sustainable superfoods into your diet not only enhances your well-being but also supports environmental stewardship. Embracing foods grown through eco-friendly practices like regenerative agriculture, crop rotation, and organic farming helps maintain soil health and biodiversity, ensuring future generations can enjoy the same nutritional benefits. Moreover, reducing food waste by creatively utilizing every part of the food—including peels, stems, and roots—maximizes nourishment and minimizes environmental impact. By consciously choosing sustainable superfoods, you contribute to a healthier planet and set a powerful example for others to follow, merging personal health with global well-being.

sustainable farming practices

Sustainable farming practices are essential for ensuring that our superfoods are both nutrient-rich and environmentally friendly. This involves using methods like crop rotation, organic farming, and permaculture to maintain soil health and reduce chemical usage. By prioritizing biodiversity, these practices help keep ecosystems balanced and resilient. Sustainable farming not only supports the Earth's natural resources but also ensures that we can continue to enjoy the health benefits of superfoods for generations to come. By choosing superfoods grown through sustainable methods, you're contributing to a healthier planet while boosting your own well-being.

Supporting Eco-Friendly Superfoods requires a shift in how we think about our food choices, not just for our own health but for the planet's well-being. Superfoods, by definition, are nutrient-dense and beneficial for our health. But it doesn't stop there. Opting for eco-friendly superfoods means choosing those that are grown using sustainable practices, minimizing harm to the environment. This dual focus on nutrition and sustainability helps us live healthier lives while contributing to a healthier planet.

Sustainable farming practices are at the heart of eco-friendly superfoods. These methods strive to balance ecological health, economic profitability, and social responsibility. Sustainable agriculture not only seeks to maintain the health of soil, water, and air but also promotes biodiversity and fair labor practices. Organic farming, crop rotation, and agroforestry are examples of practices that can produce superfoods in an environmentally friendly manner.

Organic farming is a cornerstone of sustainable agriculture. It avoids using synthetic pesticides, herbicides, and fertilizers, instead relying on natural substances and physical, mechanical, or biological methods to control pests and weeds. This practice not only produces healthier crops but also reduces harmful runoff that can contaminate water sources. By choosing organically grown superfoods like kale or blueberries, we're not just boosting our nutrient intake; we're also supporting a cleaner environment.

Crop rotation is another practice that supports eco-friendly superfoods. By rotating different crops in the same growing area, farmers can improve soil health, reduce the risk of pests and diseases, and increase biodiversity. For instance, alternating nitrogen-fixing legumes like lentils with leafy greens like spinach can naturally enrich the soil with nutrients. This practice contributes to the sustainability of farming systems while providing us with a variety of nutrient-rich foods.

Agroforestry integrates trees and shrubs into cropland and pastures. This practice can significantly enhance biodiversity, reduce erosion, and improve water retention in the soil. For example, shade-grown coffee is an agroforestry product that supports a diverse ecosystem while providing us with a nutrient-rich beverage. Encouraging the use of such methods means that we're endorsing a system that creates mutual benefits for both the environment and our health.

Local sourcing of superfoods can also contribute to their eco-friendliness. Transporting food over long distances requires significant energy, contributing to carbon emissions. By opting for locally grown superfoods, we reduce the carbon footprint associated with our consumption. Farmers' markets, community-supported agriculture (CSA) programs, and local food co-ops are excellent avenues to source superfoods like fresh berries, leafy greens, and whole grains while reducing transportation-related environmental impacts.

Reducing food waste is another crucial aspect of supporting eco-friendly superfoods. An alarming percentage of food produced for human consumption is wasted, contributing to unnecessary strain on the environment. By planning meals carefully, storing food properly, and composting organic waste, we can minimize food wastage. This not only conserves resources but also ensures that the nutrients from superfoods are fully utilized in our diets.

Water management in farming practices is critical to sustain eco-friendly superfoods. Efficient irrigation systems like drip or sprinkler irrigation can significantly reduce water usage compared to traditional methods. Additionally, selecting drought-resistant superfoods like quinoa can alleviate pressure on water resources. By supporting farms that implement these techniques, consumers can help conserve one of our planet's most precious resources.

Supporting eco-friendly superfoods also involves advocating for fair trade practices. Many superfoods, such as quinoa and chia seeds, are grown in developing countries. Fair trade certifications ensure that the farmers who cultivate these crops receive fair wages and work under safe conditions. By choosing fair trade-certified superfoods, we can help uplift communities economically while promoting ethical farming practices.

Consumers play a vital role in driving the demand for eco-friendly superfoods. As awareness about sustainable practices grows, so does the market for these products. By making informed choices and prioritizing eco-friendly superfoods, we can encourage more farmers to adopt sustainable methods. This demand shifts agricultural practices towards a more environmentally conscious model, creating a ripple effect that benefits the entire ecosystem.

Incorporating eco-friendly superfoods into daily life can be both rewarding and straightforward. Simple actions, like choosing organic berries or locally grown leafy greens, can have a significant impact. Try starting a garden to grow your own superfoods; it's a fulfilling way to ensure you're eating the freshest, most sustainably grown produce possible. Moreover, understanding labels and certifications can help you identify and select products that align with sustainable practices.

Educational initiatives can also support the eco-friendly superfood movement. Knowledge is power; by learning about the environmental impact of different farming practices, consumers are better equipped to make choices that benefit the planet. Workshops on sustainable agriculture, farm tours, and informational campaigns can bridge the gap between producers and consumers, fostering a community united by the goal of healthier living and a healthier planet.

Household changes can support eco-friendly superfoods as well. Reducing single-use plastics, using reusable bags for grocery shopping, and supporting zero-waste stores can complement the choice of eco-friendly superfoods. Kitchen practices like composting food scraps and using energy-efficient appliances further align with sustainable living. When our homes and lifestyles reflect our commitment to the environment, every meal becomes an opportunity to live our values.

In conclusion, **Supporting Eco-Friendly Superfoods** is not just about making dietary changes; it is about adopting a holistic approach that benefits personal health and the environment. By prioritizing sustainably grown, locally sourced, and fairly traded superfoods, we're making a commitment to the planet while nourishing our bodies. This harmonious approach to eating respects the earth's resources and ensures that we can enjoy the benefits of superfoods for generations to come. Together, we can cultivate a more sustainable future, one superfood at a time.

Reducing Food Waste

When it comes to sustainable superfoods, reducing food waste is a crucial piece of the puzzle. Integrating strategies like proper meal planning and creative use of leftovers can significantly cut down on waste, ensuring that every nutrient-rich ingredient finds its way to your plate and not the trash. By making small adjustments, such as shopping with a list, storing food correctly, and understanding expiration labels, you can make the most out of your superfoods. Implementing these habits doesn't just benefit your health but also contributes to a more sustainable food system, supporting both environmental and community well-being.

Tips for Optimal Food Use ... Let's dive into a part of our superfood journey that emphasizes not just what we eat, but how we use our food mindfully, ensuring nothing goes to waste. In a world where food waste is alarmingly high, implementing strategies for optimal food use can make a significant difference. Not only does it benefit our planet, but it also allows us to enjoy a wider variety of nutrient-dense foods while maximizing their health benefits.

Prioritize freshness. When you bring home a haul of superfoods, such as leafy greens, berries, and vegetables, make a plan to consume the most perishable items first. For example, spinach and berries tend to spoil faster than hardier vegetables like sweet potatoes or squash. Consuming these moisture-rich foods early ensures you get the most nutrients and flavor from your purchases.

Embrace meal prepping. By setting aside a few hours each week to wash, chop, and store your superfoods, you can streamline your cooking process and reduce waste. Use airtight containers to keep prepped ingredients fresh. For instance, kale can be washed and stripped from its stems, then stored in a container lined with a paper towel to absorb excess moisture. This makes it easy to toss into a smoothie or sauté for a quick side dish.

Another key tip is using every part of your food. Rather than discarding stems or leaves, find ways to incorporate them into your meals. Broccoli stems, for example, can be peeled, sliced, and added to stir-fries or soups. Even the leafy tops of vegetables like carrots and beets can be blended into pestos or sautéed for a nutritious side.

Explore fermentation. Fermenting vegetables not only extends their shelf life but also enhances their nutritional value. Consider fermenting excess cabbage into kimchi or sauerkraut. You can also try making your own kombucha with leftover fruit and tea. These fermented foods add probiotics to your diet, supporting gut health while ensuring zero waste.

Batch cooking can be your ally for minimizing waste and maximizing efficiency. Prepare large quantities of superfood-rich dishes, like lentil soups or quinoa salads, and portion them out for the week. This not only saves time but also ensures you have healthy meals readily available. Freeze portions you won't eat within a few days, preserving them at peak freshness.

Utilize your freezer to its full potential. If you notice fruits or vegetables nearing the end of their freshness, freeze them before they spoil. Frozen berries are perfect for smoothies, and leafy greens can be blended and portioned into ice cube trays for future use in soups and stews. Even cooked grains and legumes can be frozen, making meal prep easier on busy days.

Composting is another important aspect of optimal food use. Even with careful planning, some scraps and peelings are inevitable. Instead of sending them to the landfill, composting turns these scraps into nutrient-rich soil for your garden. This cycle of growth and regeneration benefits both your homegrown produce and the environment.

Shopping smartly is foundational to reducing waste. Make a list before heading to the grocery store, and stick to it. Purchasing only what you need for the week minimizes the risk of produce going bad. Explore bulk sections for nuts, seeds, and grains, buying just the right amount to avoid excess.

Incorporate versatile superfoods that can be used in multiple dishes. For instance, chia seeds are not only great for puddings but can also thicken jams, enrich smoothies, or be sprinkled on salads. Almonds can be enjoyed raw, made into almond butter, or used as a crunchy topping. Flexibility in your superfood selection ensures they're fully utilized.

Stock your pantry with staples that complement a variety of superfoods. Having a good selection of herbs, spices, and basic ingredients like olive oil and vinegar means you can whip up flavorful dishes without needing to constantly purchase new items. This approach helps reduce waste by enabling creative use of what you already have.

Creativity in the kitchen can minimize waste significantly. Use up veggie scraps in broths or make a "clean-out-the-fridge" stir-fry to ensure no bits are left unused. These dishes not only prevent wastage but also encourage trying new flavor combinations and cooking methods.

Mindful portioning can also play a role. Serve food in moderate portions, allowing for seconds if still hungry, rather than overloading plates initially. This reduces the amount of uneaten food that ends up in the trash. Leftovers should be promptly stored and labeled with dates to keep track of their viability.

Be aware of storage techniques to extend the freshness of superfoods. Some foods, like tomatoes and basil, are best kept at room temperature, while others, like most leafy greens and berries, should be refrigerated. Learning the optimal storage conditions for your foods can significantly prolong their usability.

Sharing surplus with neighbors or friends is another great way to ensure no food goes to waste. If you have an abundance of garden produce or bulk-bought superfoods, offering some to those around you can foster community while making the best use of your resources.

Lastly, educating yourself continuously about superfoods and their uses ensures that you remain adaptable and innovative in your approach to food. Keep an eye out for new recipes, storage hacks, and preparation tips. Knowledge is a powerful tool in reducing waste and optimizing your superfood intake.

In conclusion, using food optimally is as much about planning and preparation as it is about creativity and knowledge. By approaching your superfood consumption with mindful strategies, you not only enhance your health and well-being but also contribute to a more sustainable world. Incorporating these tips into your daily routine will help you maximize the benefits of superfoods while minimizing waste. It's a harmonious way to nurture both yourself and the planet.

Conclusion

The journey we've embarked on through the vast world of nutrient-rich superfoods has been nothing short of enlightening. We've explored a plethora of fruits, vegetables, grains, nuts, seeds, and other natural wonders that hold the potential to transform our health and longevity. By understanding and integrating these powerful ingredients into our daily lives, we've laid down a robust foundation for a healthier future.

One of the key takeaways from this exploration is the undeniable connection between what we eat and how we feel. Superfoods aren't just a trend; they're backed by science demonstrating their efficacy in boosting immunity, reducing inflammation, and providing essential nutrients. From blueberries to quinoa, from turmeric to kombucha, each superfood brings its own unique set of benefits to the table.

Incorporating superfoods into your diet doesn't have to be complicated. Simple adjustments, such as adding berries to your morning smoothie or sprinkling chia seeds over your salad, can have significant impacts on your overall well-being. These small, manageable changes, when consistently applied, can lead to lasting health benefits.

Moreover, the diverse flavors and textures of these superfoods can make your meals more enjoyable and exciting. Experimenting with new recipes, trying different cooking methods, or even just swapping out a less nutrient-dense ingredient for a superfood option can creatively and deliciously enhance your diet.

It's also important to remember the sustainability aspect of our food choices. Opting for superfoods that are grown and harvested through eco-friendly practices supports not just our health but the health of our planet. Sustainable farming practices ensure that we can continue to enjoy these foods for generations to come, while also reducing our environmental impact.

Superfoods can also be tailored to meet specific health goals. Whether you're aiming to improve heart health, manage weight, or boost energy levels, there's likely a superfood that can help you get there. The versatility of these ingredients allows for targeted nutritional strategies that can be personalized to suit individual needs.

In the hustle and bustle of modern life, quick and easy superfood snacks can provide a much-needed energy boost and nutritional support. Superfoods for kids can be a game-changer, making nutrition fun and accessible for the young ones. Engaging children with colorful, delicious superfood dishes can set them on a path of healthy eating habits that last a lifetime.

Despite the myriad benefits, it's crucial to approach superfoods with a balanced perspective. While they are incredibly beneficial, they aren't magic bullets. They work best as part of a balanced diet and a healthy lifestyle. Regular physical activity, adequate sleep, and stress management are all essential components of a holistic approach to health.

We've also dispelled some common myths and misconceptions about superfoods. It's easy to get swept up in the marketing hype, but a critical, informed approach helps us distinguish fact from fiction. Verified benefits of superfoods are well-documented, but it's important to remain discerning and cautious about exaggerated claims.

The last chapters have equipped you with practical tips for integrating superfoods into your daily life, from smart shopping strategies to efficient meal planning. By adopting these practices, you're more likely to make lasting changes that support your health goals without feeling overwhelmed.

As we bring this book to a close, it's clear that superfoods offer a versatile, effective, and enjoyable way to enhance health and longevity. The wealth of nutrients they provide can help combat chronic diseases, boost energy levels, and support overall well-being. Whether you're a seasoned health enthusiast or just beginning your journey, there are countless ways to benefit from incorporating superfoods into your diet.

The path to better health is a lifelong journey. While it may seem daunting at times, the incremental steps you take each day by choosing nutrient-rich foods will accumulate into significant, positive changes. Embrace the variety and richness that superfoods bring to your table, and let them be a cornerstone of your health journey.

Ultimately, the essence of incorporating superfoods is about empowering yourself with knowledge and making conscious choices that prioritise wellness. It's about realizing that every meal is an opportunity to nourish your body and mind. By embracing this approach, you're not just adding years to your life, but life to your years.

Thank you for embarking on this journey with us. We hope that the insights, recipes, and practical tips provided in this book inspire and empower you to make healthier choices every day. Here's to a future brimming with vitality, joy, and the incredible benefits of superfoods.

Appendix A:
Appendix

This appendix serves as a comprehensive guide to support your journey towards optimal health and longevity through the power of superfoods. It provides a quick reference to essential information, from nutrient profiles to practical tips on how to incorporate these powerhouse foods into your daily routine. Drawing from various chapters in this book, the appendix aims to synthesize key insights and actionable advice, making it easy for you to implement and sustain positive dietary changes. Whether you're looking to understand the specifics of a particular superfood, need guidance on meal planning, or want to dive deeper into the science of nutrition, this appendix is your go-to resource to ensure you're well-equipped on your path to vibrant health."

Glossary of Superfoods

Welcome to the Glossary of Superfoods, a quick reference guide for understanding the nutrient-dense foods that can enhance your health and longevity. Each entry provides a brief description of the superfood, highlighting its key benefits and typical uses.

Acai

A small, dark purple berry from the Amazon rainforest, known for its high antioxidant content and ability to boost energy levels and support overall health.

Almonds

These nutrient-rich nuts are a great source of healthy fats, protein, and fiber. They can help regulate blood sugar levels and improve heart health.

Ashwagandha

An adaptogenic herb traditionally used in Ayurvedic medicine to reduce stress and increase energy levels. Often found in powdered form, it's added to smoothies or teas.

Blueberries

These small, blue fruits are packed with antioxidants, vitamins, and fiber, making them excellent for brain and heart health.

Broccoli

A cruciferous vegetable loaded with vitamins C and K, fiber, and cancer-fighting compounds. It can be enjoyed steamed, roasted, or raw.

Chia Seeds

These tiny seeds are rich in omega-3 fatty acids, fiber, and protein. They help in digestion and can be easily added to puddings, smoothies, and baked goods.

Chickpeas

A versatile legume high in protein and fiber, chickpeas are great for supporting digestive health and can be used in salads, stews, and hummus.

Dark Chocolate

Rich in antioxidants and flavonoids, dark chocolate supports heart health. Opt for varieties with at least 70% cocoa content for maximum benefits.

Ginger

This spicy root is known for its anti-inflammatory properties and ability to aid digestion. It's often added to teas, soups, and stir-fries.

Goji Berries

Also known as "red diamonds," these berries are high in antioxidants and believed to enhance immune function and promote eye health.

Kale

A leafy green superfood, kale is loaded with vitamins A, C, and K, as well as minerals and antioxidants. It's great in salads, soups, and smoothies.

Kelp

This edible seaweed is a fantastic source of iodine, essential for thyroid function, and offers a range of minerals and vitamins.

Kefir

A fermented dairy product rich in probiotics, kefir supports gut health and digestion. It can be consumed on its own or added to smoothies and cereals.

Lemons

Loaded with vitamin C, lemons are great for detoxification and boosting the immune system. They can be used in drinks, dressings, and marinades.

Lentils

High in protein, fiber, and essential nutrients, lentils are excellent for heart health and can be used in soups, salads, and stews.

Maca

A root vegetable from the Andes, maca is known for its energy-boosting properties. It's commonly available in powder form and added to smoothies.

Nori

A type of seaweed used in sushi, nori is rich in vitamins and minerals, particularly iodine, which supports thyroid function.

Olive Oil

Known as "liquid gold," this healthy fat is rich in monounsaturated fats and antioxidants. It's great for heart health and is used in cooking and dressings.

Pomegranate

This ancient superfood is packed with antioxidants and vitamins, promoting heart health and reducing inflammation. Enjoy the seeds fresh or as juice.

Quinoa

A gluten-free whole grain that's a complete protein, quinoa is loaded with fiber, vitamins, and minerals. Ideal for salads, bowls, and side dishes.

Reishi Mushroom

Also known as the "mushroom of immortality," reishi is famed for boosting the immune system and reducing stress. It's often consumed in tinctures or teas.

Spinach

A leafy green rich in iron, calcium, and vitamins A and C. Spinach supports bone health and boosts immunity, perfect for salads, soups, and smoothies.

Strawberries

These red berries are high in vitamin C, manganese, and antioxidants, making them great for skin health and reducing inflammation.

Sweet Potatoes

Rich in vitamins A and C, fiber, and complex carbohydrates, sweet potatoes support eye health and provide lasting energy. They can be roasted, mashed, or added to soups.

Turmeric

Known for its powerful anti-inflammatory and antioxidant properties, turmeric is widely used in cooking and as a supplement for its health benefits.

Wild Salmon

A rich source of omega-3 fatty acids, high-quality protein, and essential vitamins, wild salmon supports heart and brain health. It can be grilled, baked, or broiled.

This glossary serves as a quick reference to the myriad of superfoods that can boost your health. To dive deeper into the benefits and uses of these nutrient powerhouses, explore the corresponding chapters of this book.

Additional Resources for Health and Longevity

In an era where the quest for health and longevity is more pressing than ever, finding reliable and scientifically-backed resources becomes crucial. While this book provides a comprehensive guide to superfoods and their benefits, continuing your education through additional references can ensure a deeper understanding and more effective application of these nutrient powerhouses in your daily life. Below is a compilation of various resources that can enrich your knowledge about superfoods and their role in health and longevity.

To start with, numerous academic journals publish cutting-edge research on nutrition and superfoods. Journals such as the "Journal of Nutrition," "American Journal of Clinical Nutrition," and "Food & Function" regularly explore the biochemical properties of superfoods and their impacts on health. These journals are peer-reviewed, ensuring the credibility of the information presented and are an excellent way to stay updated on the latest scientific advancements.

Books are another valuable source of information. For those fascinated by the intricate relationship between food and health, consider exploring titles dedicated to specific superfoods or nutritional science. Books often provide in-depth insights, combining historical contexts, up-to-date research, and practical tips. They offer a broader perspective that can be beneficial for anyone looking to dig deeper into the subject.

Online courses and webinars also present an effective way to expand your knowledge. Platforms like Coursera, Udemy, and even some universities offer courses specifically focused on nutrition and superfoods. These courses range from beginner to advanced levels, covering various aspects from the basic nutritional content to advanced integration into meal planning. Webinars often feature experts in the field who provide insights, answer questions, and share the latest trends.

Podcasts and video series are fantastic resources for those who prefer auditory and visual learning. Channels like YouTube feature numerous nutritionists and dietitians who discuss superfoods and offer practical tips for incorporating them into daily meals. Podcasts hosted by industry experts often delve into current trends, debates, and success stories, making them an engaging way to stay informed while multitasking.

Social media platforms can be surprisingly useful for discovering new recipes, tips, and the latest research. Follow reputable nutritionists, dietitians, and health-focused chefs who share effective ways to incorporate superfoods into everyday life. Platforms such as Instagram and Pinterest offer visual inspiration through photos and step-by-step guides, making it easier to understand and try out new superfood-rich recipes.

Joining local or online communities focused on health and nutrition can offer the added benefit of peer support. These communities are often rich in shared experiences, recommendations, and encouragement, which can be particularly motivating. Local farmer's markets and health food stores frequently host events and workshops that can provide hands-on experience with superfoods.

Additionally, government health sites, such as the National Institutes of Health (NIH) and the Centers for Disease Control and Prevention (CDC), offer trustworthy information on nutrition and health. These sites frequently update their databases with articles, studies, and guidelines that can help you understand the official perspective on dietary recommendations and how superfoods fit into the larger picture of health.

For insights specifically geared towards holistic health, natural health magazines and journals often focus on the broad spectrum of benefits provided by superfoods, including their role in alternative medicine. Publications such as "Wellness" and "Alternative Medicine Review" explore the traditional uses and modern applications of various superfoods, adding another layer to your understanding.

Cooking apps and digital recipe platforms such as Yummly and Epicurious can be handy tools. These platforms allow you to filter recipes based on specific superfoods and dietary needs. They often feature user reviews, making it easier to find tried-and-tested recipes that fit into your lifestyle seamlessly.

Finally, consulting with healthcare professionals provides personalized guidance tailored to your unique health needs and goals. Dietitians, nutritionists, and even doctors can offer specialized advice on how to integrate superfoods into your diet effectively. Personalized nutrition plans and consultations ensure that your superfood consumption is not just healthy, but optimal for your individual requirements.

By leveraging these additional resources, you can enrich your understanding and practical use of superfoods, ensuring that your journey towards enhanced health and longevity is both informed and effective. Each resource offers a unique perspective and piece of the puzzle, contributing to a holistic approach to wellness.

www.ingramcontent.com/pod-product-compliance
Lightning Source LLC
Chambersburg PA
CBHW030310290526
45785CB00001B/289